ESSENTI

ESSENTIAL HISTOLOGY REVIEW

FRANK J.WILSON, PhD
Department of Neuroscience and Cell Biology
University of Medicine and Dentistry of New Jersey
Robert Wood Johnson Medical School

JEAN A. GIBNEY, BA
Department of Neuroscience and Cell Biology
University of Medicine and Dentistry of New Jersey
Robert Wood Johnson Medical School

SHANNON G. MATTA, PhD
Endocrine Neuroscience Laboratories
Minneapolis Medical Research Foundation
Department of Medicine
Hennepin County Medical Center and the University of Minnesota

MATTHEW G. KESTENBAUM, MD
Department of Internal Medicine
Northwestern Memorial Hospital

b

Blackwell
Science

BLACKWELL SCIENCE

EDITORIAL OFFICES:
238 Main Street, Cambridge, Massachusetts 02142, USA
Osney Mead, Oxford OX2 0E1, England
25 John Street, London WC1N 2BL, England
23 Ainslie Place, Edinburgh EH3 6AJ, Scotland
54 University Street, Carlton, Victoria 3053, Australia
Arnette Blackwell SA, 1 rue de Lille, 75007 Paris, France
Blackwell Wissenschafts-Verlag GmbH Kurfürstendamm 57, 10707 Berlin, Germany
Feldgasse 13, A-1238 Vienna, Austria

DISTRIBUTORS:

USA
Blackwell Science, Inc.
238 Main Street
Cambridge, Massachusetts 02142
(Telephone orders: 800-215-1000 or 617-876-7000)

Canada
Copp Clark, Ltd.
2775 Matheson Blvd. East
Mississauga, Ontario
Canada, L4W 4P7
(Telephone orders: 800-263-4374 or 905-238-6074)

Australia
Blackwell Science Pty., Ltd.
54 University Street
Carlton, Victoria 3053
(Telephone orders: 03-9347-0300
Fax 03-9349-3016)

Outside North America and Australia
Blackwell Science, Ltd.
c/o Marston Book Services, Ltd.
P.O. Box 87
Oxford OX2 0DT
England
(Telephone orders: 44-1865-791155)

Acquisitions: Joy Denomme
Development: Kathleen Broderick
Production: Heather Garrison
Manufacturing: Karen Feeney
Typeset by Dartmouth Publishing, Inc.
Printed and bound by DS Graphics

Printed in the United States of America
96 97 98 99 5 4 3 2 1

Library of Congress Cataloging-in-Publication Data

Essential histology review / Frank J. Wilson . . . [et al.].
  p. cm.
Includes bibliographical references and index.
ISBN 0-86542-487-x (alk. paper)
1. Histology—Examinations, questions, etc.   I. Wilson, Frank J.
(Frank Joseph), 1941–
QM554.E85 1996   96-1559
611'.018' 076—dc20   CIP

CONTENTS

PREFACE

A course in histology should not necessitate the students' memorization of illustrated material and associated questions. Histology is a complex subject that requires an organized approach to the microscopic recognition of tissue and a strong knowledge base regarding the structure and function of that tissue. We have compiled over 500 questions arranged in twenty chapters beginning with Methods of Histology and concluding with Organs of Special Sense. Several light and electron micrographs have been included as part of the multiple choice questions. The questions range from those that are quite challenging to those that are rather straightforward. The authors hope that by careful review of each question and its accompanying Learning Response students will develop a framework for approaching the subject matter that is based on understanding rather than memorization. This strategy should prove helpful in preparation for both course examinations and board examinations.

The authors thank Mary Jo Norris for providing some of the electron micrographs included in this publication. In addition, we are indebted to Cheryl Dreyfus, Sarah Hitchcock-DeGregori, Gordon Macdonald and W. Geoffrey McAuliffe who, as faculty teaching in the Cell Biology and Histology course at Robert Wood Johnson Medical School, continually provide students with stimulating examination questions. We are deeply grateful for the love and support of our spouses and children, Alfreda, Frank and Lynda Wilson, John, Jillian, Jocelyn and Jason, Brandi and grandson Sean Gibney, John and Megan Matta and Kathleen Fink-Kestenbaum without whom life would have little meaning. Lastly, we thank those individuals who taught us histology: Melvin Hess, Philip Krutzsch, and Albert Lansing formerly of the University of Pittsburgh School of Medicine, Bruce Babiarz of Rutgers University and Anna-Mary Carpenter formerly of the University of Minnesota School of Medicine. Their enthusiasm for, and devotion to, the subject of histology have been an inspiration to us who now carry on their traditions and examples.

FJW
JAG
SGM
MGK

1. SUBJECT AREA: Methods in Histology
QUESTION: The resolution of the light microscope is approximately

A: one micrometer.
B: 0.2 micrometers.
C: 0.5 micrometers.
D: one nanometer.
E: 100 angstrom units.

Learning Response B: Correct. The highest resolution of the best light microscopes is approximately 0.2 micrometers.

2. SUBJECT AREA: Methods in Histology
QUESTION: Injection of radioactive substances into cells allows researchers to study

A: the synthesis of DNA.
B: the metabolism of carbohydrates.
C: intracellular pathways of secretion.
D: the fate of intracellular lipid.
E: all of the above cellular processes.

Learning Response E: Correct. A wide variety of cellular activities can be studied with radioactive precursors.

3. SUBJECT AREA: Methods in Histology
QUESTION: Differences between light and electron microscopes include all of the following EXCEPT

A: the light microscope requires a fluorescent screen to view the specimen.
B: the electron microscope requires extremely thin specimens.
C: the electron microscope requires heavy metals to enhance contrast of the specimen.

D: both use a condenser lens to focus the beam of illumination.

E: the electron microscope uses a beam of electrons to examine the specimen.

Learning Response A: Correct. Specimens viewed with the light microscope can be examined by peering through the oculars or by photographing the image with an attached camera.

4.   SUBJECT AREA: Methods in Histology

QUESTION: The units of measurement called Angstrom and micron have been replaced by

A: centimeter and millimeter.
B: nanometer and millimeter.
C: nanometer and centimeter.
D: nanometer and micrometer.
E: micrometer and nanometer.

Learning Response D: Correct. The unit of measure called Angstrom has been replaced by nanometer (10^{-9} meter); one nanometer = 10 Angstroms. The unit called micron is now termed micrometer and corresponds to 10^{-6} meter.

5.   SUBJECT AREA: Methods in Histology

QUESTION: An acidophilic structure within a cell or tissue

A: repels acid dyes.
B: attracts acid dyes.
C: stains with basic dyes.
D: stains equally with acid or basic dyes.
E: exhibits none of the above features.

Learning Response B: Correct. Acidophilia is a property associated with cells, tissues and organs and refers to the affinity of material in the cell, tissue or organ for acidic dyes such as eosin.

6. SUBJECT AREA: Methods in Histology
QUESTION: Lipids are best demonstrated by reacting with

A: silver nitrate dyes.
B: hematoxylin and eosin.
C: periodic acid-Schiff (PAS) reagent.
D: Sudan dyes.
E: Feulgen stain.

Learning Response D: Correct. Lipids are best visualized with dyes that are lipid soluble. Sudan IV and Sudan black impart red and black colors, respectively, on lipids.

7. SUBJECT AREA: Methods in Histology
QUESTION: Polysaccharides such as glycogen and glycosaminoglycans are best demonstrated by reaction with

A: hematoxylin and eosin.
B: periodic acid-Schiff (PAS) reagent.
C: Sudan black.
D: acid phosphatase reaction.
E: alkaline phosphatase reaction.

Learning Response B: Correct. Intracellular, plasma membrane bound and extracellular polysaccharides can be stained with PAS.

8. SUBJECT AREA: Methods in Histology
QUESTION: The basis for immunocytochemical reactions is

A: the affinity of an antigen for its homologous antibody.
B: the localization of radioactive precursors.
C: the affinity of acidophilic substances for eosin.
D: the detection of acid phosphatase reactions.
E: the detection of acridine orange complexes.

Learning Response A: Correct. Antigenic substances in cells and tissues can be identified by the reaction of its antibody which has been conjugated with either a fluorescent dye, enzyme or gold particles.

9. SUBJECT AREA: Methods in Histology
     QUESTION In the indirect antibody labeling method,

    A: the fluorescent dye is coupled to the antigen.
    B: the primary antibody directed against the antigen is labeled.
    C: a secondary antibody is labeled and this antibody reacts with the primary antibody.
    D: an enzyme such as peroxidase is used to label the primary antibody.
    E: neither antigens nor antibodies are labeled and heavy metal stains are reacted with the antigen-antibody complexes.

Learning Response C: Correct. The labeled secondary antibody marks the location of the primary antibody which marks the location of the antigen in the cell or tissue forming the basis of the indirect immunocytochemical method.

10. SUBJECT AREA: Methods in Histology
     QUESTION: Which technique would be best for studying the distribution of proteins in a membrane?

    A: transmission electron microscopy of a sectioned specimen
    B: scanning electron microscopy
    C: freeze fracture
    D: indirect immunofluorescence
    E: periodic acid-Schiff (PAS) staining

Learning Response C: Correct. Freeze fracture demonstrates the arrangement of proteins in the membrane leaflets.

11. SUBJECT AREA: Methods in Histology

QUESTION: The hydrogen peroxide and 3,3'-diaminoazobenzidine (DAB) method is the most commonly used technique because

A: it is readily available commercially.

B: it can be used for diagnostic purposes as well as a label in immunocytochemistry and hybridization techniques.

C: it is an inexpensive method to use.

D: the substrate can be dissolved out of the tissue allowing for another type of stain to be applied to the same tissue.

E: it can measure the concentration of a substance by the intensity of the reaction product.

Learning Response B: Correct. The DAB method can be used in the diagnosis of leukemias by being able to detect differences in peroxidase activity in blood cells. The enzyme activity produces a substantial amount of insoluble precipitate in a very short time, making this procedure a very sensitive histochemical assay.

12. SUBJECT AREA: Methods in Histology

QUESTION: What method would best be used if you were interested in knowing if rat ovaries contained DNA specific for the gene that encodes for nerve growth factor (NGF)?

A: Southern analysis

B: Northern analysis

C: Western analysis

D: Feulgen reaction

E: DAB method

Learning Response A: Correct. Southern analysis characterizes and quantitates the presence of DNA of a specific gene in eukaryotic organisms. Northern analysis identifies and quantitates messenger RNA, and Western analysis detects proteins.

13. SUBJECT AREA: Methods in Histology

QUESTION: A Northern analysis indicates that messenger RNA for epinephrine is present in mutant adrenal medullary cells. Which one of the following methods would *best* be used to indicate the concentration of the catecholamine that is being produced?

A: immunofluorescence
B: immunocytochemistry
C: hematoxylin and eosin
D: fluorescence spectroscopy
E: *in situ* hybridization

Learning Response D: Correct. Western analysis detects and quantifies specific proteins found in cells. Immunocytochemistry and immunofluorescence are able to localize the protein within the tissue, but it would not be able to give accurate quantities of protein found within the tissue. *In situ* hybridization is a semiquantitative technique and the presence of messenger RNA does not always correlate with protein. The study of catecholamines by fluorescent probes would probably be the best choice.

14. SUBJECT AREA: Methods in Histology

QUESTION: In reference to *in situ* hybridization, probes can be

A: proteins labeled with fluorescent tags.
B: labeled complementary DNA sequences.
C: antibodies conjugated to gold particles
D: fine instruments used to perforate cell membranes to allow for DNA transfection.
E: restriction enzymes used to break up DNA.

Learning Response B: Correct. Probes are known labeled complementary single-stranded nucleic acid sequences. They are usually labeled with radioisotopes or biotin.

15. SUBJECT AREA: Methods in Histology

QUESTION: Lysosomes within cells can be identified by using

A: acid phosphatase reactions.
B: the Feulgen reaction.
C: osmium.
D: hematoxylin and eosin.
E: periodic acid-Schiff (PAS) reaction.

Learning Response A: Correct. Lysosomes are cytoplasmic organelles that contain the enzyme *acid phosphatase,* the presence of which can be used to identify lysosomes. Cells are incubated in a solution containing sodium glycerophosphate and lead nitrate buffered to pH 5.0. Acid phosphatase hydrolyzes the glycerophosphate, liberating phosphate ions. These ions react with lead nitrate to produce an insoluble, colorless precipitate of lead phosphate at the specific site of the enzymatic activity. In order to visualize this reaction, the cells are immersed in a solution of ammonium sulfide which will react with the lead phosphate to produce a black precipitate of lead sulfide. Lead sulfide is opaque and can be seen in the electron microscope.

---

16.   SUBJECT AREA: Cytology
      QUESTION: Which of the following structures is NOT bound by a membrane?

      A: cilia
      B: lipid droplets
      C: mitochondria
      D: secretory granules
      E: lysosomes

Learning Response B: Correct. A trilaminar cell membrane encloses all of the above except lipid droplets which are located in the cytosol.

---

17.   SUBJECT AREA: Cytology
      QUESTION: Which of the following mitotic processes would be inhibited by microinjection of antibodies to nonmuscle myosin?

      A: centriole movements to opposite poles

> *B:* cytokinesis
> *C:* chromosome movements at anaphase
> *D:* formation of the spindle apparatus
> *E:* disappearance of the nucleolus in prophase

Learning Response B: Correct. In telophase, a constriction develops in the parent cell and progresses until it divides the cytoplasm. The presence of both actin and myosin are necessary for this process called cytokinesis.

---

18. SUBJECT AREA: Cytology
       QUESTION: Which of the following classes of intermediate filaments is found in muscle cells?

> *A:* vimentin filaments
> *B:* cytokeratin filaments
> *C:* desmin filaments
> *D:* myosin filaments
> *E:* tonofilaments

Learning Response C: Correct. Desmin is associated with the intermediate filaments in the three types of muscle. Vimentin filaments are found in cells originating from mesenchyme. Cytokeratin filaments are located in epithelial cells. Myosin filaments are classified as contractile and are not intermediate filaments. Tonofilaments are classified as cytokeratin filament types in epithelial cells.

---

19. SUBJECT AREA: Cytology
       QUESTION: Nuclear pores

> *A:* allow macromolecules to pass to and from the nucleolus.
> *B:* are studded with ribosomes.
> *C:* are blocked by heterochromatin.
> *D:* are morphologically similar to communicating (gap) junctions.
> *E:* allow macromolecules to pass to and from the cytoplasm.

Learning Response E: Correct. Nuclear pores provide passageway for molecules into and out of the nucleus. The outer membrane of the nuclear envelope has ribosomes associated with it, but these structures do not extend into the nuclear pores. In the vicinity of nuclear pores inside the nucleus heterochromatin is absent. Communicating junctions can exist as extensive areas of the surfaces of two cells, and a small gap of extracellular space can be seen between the cells.

---

20. SUBJECT AREA: Cytology

QUESTION: Which of the following is necessary for the nuclear envelope to break down during mitosis?

A: phosphorylation of nuclear lamins
B: duplication of the centrioles
C: formation of the mitotic spindle
D: condensation of chromosomes
E: migration of chromosomes to the equatorial plate

Learning Response A: Correct. Nuclear lamins are a class of intermediate filament proteins which form a network just under the nuclear envelope as part of a structure called the fibrous lamina. Phosphorylation of these proteins is the key event in the disintegration of the nuclear envelope in mitosis.

---

21. SUBJECT AREA: Cytology

QUESTION: Electron micrographs of cilia of patients with a genetic disease called immotile cilia syndrome reveal an absence of the outer dynein arms and the presence of abnormal single microtubules. What are the consequences of this defective structure?

A: If the patient is a male, swimming movements of spermatozoa would be unimpaired.
B: Mucus would accumulate in the respiratory passages which are lined by ciliated epithelium.
C: The ability of dynein to hydrolyze GTP would be impaired.
D: Anterograde movement of vesicles most likely would be impaired.

E: Isolated axonemes would probably have a normal function.

Learning Response B: Correct. The actions of the ciliated epithelium of the respiratory system would be affected by the disease. Spermatozoan movements would be impaired, but anterograde axonal transport requires kinesin, not dynein.

---

22. SUBJECT AREA: Cytology
QUESTION: Intermediate filaments

A: are not affected by phosphorylation.
B: and their associated proteins are important in determining the shape of cells.
C: are composed of a single class of proteins.
D: are one of the components of band desmosomes (zonula adherens).
E: are present only in fully differentiated cells such as neurons and skeletal muscle cells.

Learning Response B: Correct. Intermediate filaments (IF) are composed of different classes of proteins, and at least five classes have been identified. These are present in most eukaryotic cells. Phosphorylation is important in the function of IF proteins, especially the lamins of the nucleus. Actin microfilaments are associated with belt desmosomes.

---

23. SUBJECT AREA: Cytology
QUESTION: Proteins synthesized on membrane-bound polyribosomes normally may undergo each of the following EXCEPT

A: intracellular transport in vesicles.
B: release from polyribosomes into the cytosol.
C: secretion.
D: retention in the Golgi complex.
E: transfer to the lumen of the endoplasmic reticulum.

Learning Response B: Correct. Proteins of the cytosol, nucleus, peroxisomes and most mitochondrial proteins are synthesized on polysomes in the cytosol. All other intracellular and secreted proteins can be found in the endoplasmic reticulum, transport vesicles and the Golgi complex.

---

24. SUBJECT AREA: Cytology

QUESTION: A cell you are studying has condensed chromosomes, two centrosomes each with a centriole pair, and an intact nuclear envelope. What stage of the cell cycle is it in?

  A: metaphase
  B: anaphase
  C: prophase
  D: telophase
  E: interphase

Learning Response C: Correct. In mitotic prophase the nuclear envelope has not yet begun to disintegrate and the chromosomes have commenced coiling.

---

25. SUBJECT AREA: Cytology

QUESTION: What feature(s) of the plasma membrane contribute(s) to the difference between the extracellular and cytosolic surfaces?

  A: Extracellular location of glycosylated domains (regions) of membrane proteins
  B: Amphipathic character of membrane lipids
  C: Distribution of glycolipids and phospholipids
  D: Choices *A* and *B* above
  E: Choices *A* and *C* above

Learning Response E: Correct. The external location of the carbohydrate components of membrane proteins and lipids contributes to the asymmetry of the plasma membrane.

26. SUBJECT AREA: Cytology

QUESTION: When a receptor-ligand complex is internalized in a vesicle and carried to the early endosome (a vesicular compartment of the cell, pH 6.0-6.5), all of the following are possible fates of the membrane and contents of the vesicle EXCEPT

A: recycling to the plasmalemma.
B: exocytosis.
C: transcellular transport or transcytosis.
D: transfer to the Golgi complex.
E: degradation by lysosomes.

Learning Response B: Correct. Exocytosis is the process by which a membrane bound secretory vesicle fuses with the plasma membrane and the contents of the vesicle are deposited into the extracellular matrix. Transcytosis is the process by which an endosome and its contents move from one cell surface to another. This phenomenon is often seen in capillary endothelial cells or in cells that transport ions.

27. SUBJECT AREA:. Cytology

QUESTION: All of the following structures or proteins listed below, or their precursors or products, would, *at some time*, be found in the same structure, organelle or location EXCEPT

A: histones and lamin.
B: histones and actin.
C: lysosomal enzymes and ingested bacterium.
D: collagen and clathrin.
E: signal recognition peptide (SRP) receptor and low density lipoprotein (LDL) receptor.

Learning Response D: Correct. Procollagen, the precursor molecule of extracellular collagen, is synthesized on the rough endoplasmic reticulum. Clathrin is a cytosolic protein and would be synthesized on polyribosomes in the cytosol. Histones and lamin reside in the nucleus. Histones and actin would be synthesized in the cytosol. The SRP and LDL receptors would be synthesized on the rough endoplasmic reticulum.

28. SUBJECT AREA: Cytology

QUESTION: Antibody induced patching of membrane proteins and redistribution of proteins in the membrane

A: illustrate that membrane proteins can move laterally in the plane of the membrane.

B: illustrate that proteins can flip-flop across the plane of the membrane.

C: prove that certain membrane proteins are anchored to the cytoskeleton.

D: prove that the plasma membrane is a lipid bilayer.

E: require energy from the hydrolysis of ATP.

Learning Response A: Correct. The fluidity of the plasma membrane allows for the movement of receptors and other proteins within the plane of the membrane. Molecules cannot flip from one leaflet of the lipid bilayer to the other. This fluid mosaic model does not require energy for the redistribution of the membrane proteins.

29. SUBJECT AREA: Cytology

QUESTION: Movement of cilia is directly attributable to the presence of

A: myosin.

B: actin.

C: kinesin.

D: dynein.

E: cytokeratin.

Learning Response D: Correct. The motor protein or mechanochemical enzyme associated with the microtubules of cilia is dynein which has the ability to hydrolyze ATP. Myosin and actin are located in eukaryotic cells, the latter in microfilaments. Kinesin is a motor protein that functions in vesicle translocations in the cell along microtubules. In neurons, kinesin moves vesicles away from the cell body and into the neuronal cytoplasmic extensions.

30. Subject Area: Cytology

Question: Features of cells especially active in protein synthesis include all of the following EXCEPT

A: the presence of a Golgi complex.
B: a prominent nucleolus.
C: stacks of rough endoplasmic reticulum.
D: a basophilic cytoplasm.
E: an abundance of smooth endoplasmic reticulum.

Learning Response E: Correct. Cells with a large amount of smooth endoplasmic reticulum normally function in steroidogenesis.

31. Subject Area: Cytology

Question: All of the following processes would be inhibited by treatment of a cell with a drug that disrupts microtubules [Colcemid (colchicine) or Vinca alkaloids (vincristine)] EXCEPT

A: movement of chromosomes to spindle poles.
B: maintenance of cell polarity.
C: cytokinesis.
D: organization of the endoplasmic reticulum within the cell.
E: movement of vesicles from the rough endoplasmic reticulum to the Golgi.

Learning Response C: Correct. Cytokinesis, the division of one cell into two daughter cells, involves the interaction of myosin and actin, not microtubules.

32. Subject Area:. Cytology

Question: All of the following are characteristic of mitochondria EXCEPT that they

A: contain DNA.
B: exhibit a high turnover rate of their constituent enzymes.

C: can synthesize proteins.

D: serve as a storage site for glycogen.

E: contain respiratory and phosphorylation enzyme systems bound to crista membranes.

Learning Response D: Correct. Glycogen is stored in granules in the cytosol.

---

33. SUBJECT AREA: Cytology
QUESTION: The nucleolus

A: is the site of ribosomal RNA synthesis.

B: synthesizes ribosomal proteins.

C: is absent in cells actively secreting proteins.

D: is the area of the nucleus lacking DNA.

E: assembles ribosomal subunits into mature ribosomes which are transported from the nucleus.

Learning Response A: Correct. All protein synthesis occurs in the cytoplasm. Ribosomal proteins enter the nucleus and nucleolus where they are combined with ribosomal RNA transcribed from nucleolar organizer DNA. Ribosomal subunits migrate from the nucleus and are assembled on messenger RNA molecules to begin the process of protein synthesis. The nucleolus is particularly prominent in cells actively synthesizing proteins.

---

34. SUBJECT AREA: Cytology
QUESTION: A somatic cell in the late G2 stage of the cell cycle

A: has a normal diploid amount of DNA.

B: has two centrosomes (centriole replication has occurred).

C: has paired homologous chromosomes.

D: is in the longest stage of the cell cycle.

E: has not yet synthesized the tubulin needed for incorporation into the mitotic spindle.

Learning Response B: Correct. The G2 stage occurs after DNA replication (the S phase) and is the shortest phase of the cell cycle. The replication of the centrioles creates two cell centers or centrosomes, and tubulin synthesis has commenced. The chromatin is not condensed in G2.

35. SUBJECT AREA: Cytology
     QUESTION: Euchromatin

> *A:* is active in transcription.
> *B:* actively translates RNA.
> *C:* amounts are related to protein synthetic activity.
> *D:* consists of DNA without associated histones.
> *E:* appears as dense, coarse granules by electron microscopy.

Learning Response A: Correct. Actively transcribed DNA is associated with euchromatin; histone proteins are attached to euchromatin. Heterochromatin is denser than euchromatin and can be distinguished from it in electron micrographs. A cell with a large amount of euchromatin (a neuron, for example) has a large amount of its DNA being actively transcribed. A cell with an abundance of heterochromatin (a plasma cell, for example) has little of its DNA transcribed into RNA. Both are actively synthesizing proteins. The plasma cell, however, is specialized in the synthesis and secretion of a specific type of protein (immunoglobulins) while the neuron makes a wide variety of proteins.

36. SUBJECT AREA: Cytology
     QUESTION: Proteins sent to the trans Golgi network have all of the following possible destinations EXCEPT

> *A:* secretory vesicles.
> *B:* lysosomes.
> *C:* plasma membrane.
> *D:* peroxisomes.
> *E:* retention in the Golgi itself.

Learning Response D: Correct. The proteins found in the cytosol, nucleus, peroxisomes and the cytoskeleton are synthesized on polysomes in the cytosol, and not on the rough endoplasmic reticulum (RER). The proteins destined for all the other above choices are transported from the RER via transport vesicles to the Golgi and are sorted in the trans Golgi network.

---

37. SUBJECT AREA: Cytology

QUESTION: Actin is located in, or associated with all of the following structures EXCEPT

A: cytoplasmic extensions involved in cell migration.
B: the cell plate or cleavage furrow in mitosis.
C: flagella.
D: the apical cytoplasm of columnar epithelial cells.
E: in association with the thin filaments of muscle cells.

Learning Response C: Correct. Flagellar motility is based on the movements of microtubules and the interaction of the motor protein dynein with tubulin. Actin is not located in flagella.

---

38. SUBJECT AREA: Cytology

QUESTION: Which of the following features are common between mitochondria and one or more other organelles?

A: protein synthesis
B: DNA synthesis
C: RNA synthesis
D: enclosed by two membranes
E: all of the above choices

Learning Response E: Correct. Mitochondria are complex organelles and share a number of features in common with other cellular structures and with prokaryotic organisms.

---

39. SUBJECT AREA: Cytology

QUESTION: Endocytosis, in contrast to exocytosis,

A: requires membrane fusion.
B: nvolves traffic to and from the Golgi complex.

C: may be constitutive or regulated.

D: is a mechanism for transport of macromolecules across the plasmalemma.

E: can occur at clathrin coated pits.

Learning Response E: Correct. Endocytosis and exocytosis share all of the above features except the requirement for clathrin coated pits. Clathrin and its association with vesicles and invaginations of the plasma membrane (clathrin coated pits) assist in the process of receptor mediated endocytosis in which a ligand binding to its receptor is taken into the cell.

---

40. SUBJECT AREA: Cytology

QUESTION: All of the following statements are correct in reference to the endoplasmic reticulum EXCEPT

A: the smooth endoplasmic reticulum (SER) and rough endoplasmic reticulum (RER) are two independent organelles.

B: the perinuclear space of the nuclear envelope is continuous with the lumen of the RER.

C: transporting vesicles which shuttle proteins from the RER to the Golgi are part of the SER.

D: in certain organs the SER functions to detoxify noxious substances.

E: posttranslational modifications, such as glycosylation, hydroxylation, etc., of proteins can occur in the lumen of the RER.

Learning Response A: Correct. The endoplasmic reticulum is one continuous organelle as evidenced by the fact that an enzyme, glucose-6-phosphatase, is a constituent of the membranes of both the RER and SER.

---

41. SUBJECT AREA: Cytology

QUESTION: All of the following are features of peroxisomes or microbodies EXCEPT

A: the presence of crystalline inclusions.

B: their function in fatty acid oxidation.

C: all proteins are synthesized on polyribosomes in
the cytosol.

D: that they are Golgi-derived organelles.

E: for the presence of catalase which breaks down
hydrogen peroxide into water and oxygen.

Learning Response D: Correct. The proteins found in peroxisomes are
synthesized in the cytoplasm outside of the rough endoplasmic reticulum (in
the cytosol). As such the proteins that are contained in peroxisomes do not
pass through the Golgi complex.

---

42. SUBJECT AREA: Cytology

QUESTION: All of the following events occur in the synthesis of
proteins which are secreted EXCEPT

A: interruption of synthesis by the attachment of a
signal recognition peptide (SRP) to the nascent
peptide chain.

B: binding of the SRP to a receptor in the membrane
of the rough endoplasmic reticulum (RER).

C: removal of the signal peptide sequence in the
cytosol.

D: attachment of ribosomes to integral membrane
proteins in the RER.

E: initiation of protein synthesis in the cytosol.

Learning Response C: Correct. The signal peptide is removed from the
growing peptide chain by a specific enzyme located on the inner surface of
the membrane of the RER. Translation of the protein continues, and
secondary and tertiary structural changes as well as posttranslational
modifications occur intracisternally.

---

43. SUBJECT AREA: Cytology

QUESTION: Lipofuscin

A: accumulates in cells that are long-lived, such as
neurons and cardiac muscle cells.

> *B:* refers to residual bodies which remain in the cytoplasm.
> *C:* consists of membrane bound vacuoles of material resistant to lysosomal degradation.
> *D:* is characterized by choices A and B above.
> *E:* has features described in choices A, B and C above.

Learning Response E: Correct. Lipofuscin which is also known as age pigment accumulates in cells as large quantities of residual bodies. The material enclosed in the cell membrane is the undigested products of lysosomal enzyme activity.

44. SUBJECT AREA: Cytology
QUESTION: During its synthesis and transport, the *cytosolic domain* (region) of a transmembrane protein destined for the plasma membrane may be found at which of the following locations.

> *A:* Luminal surface of the endoplasmic reticulum
> *B:* Cytosolic surface of transport (transfer) vesicles
> *C:* Attached to free ribosomes in the cytosol
> *D:* As part of a free protein in the cytosol
> *E:* Luminal surface of cisternae in the Golgi apparatus

Learning Response B: Correct. Membrane proteins are synthesized on the rough endoplasmic reticulum, transported to the Golgi complex and targeted to the plasma membrane. The cytosolic domain of the protein would be found on the cytosolic surface of transport vesicles which shuttle protein from the endoplasmic reticulum to the Golgi.

45. SUBJECT AREA:. Cytology
QUESTION: An interphase cell in G1 contains a pair of most chromosomes. How many *strands* (polynucleotide chains) of DNA are in each pair?

> *A:* 1
> *B:* 2
> *C:* 4

D: 8
E: 46

Learning Response C: Correct. Each chromosome contains one DNA molecule composed of two polynucleotide chains. Since there is a pair of chromosomes in the cell at G1, prior to the S phase of the cell cycle when DNA replication occurs, there would be four polynucleotide chains of DNA in each pair.

---

46. SUBJECT AREA: Cytology
QUESTION: Identify the structures indicated by the arrows in the figure below.

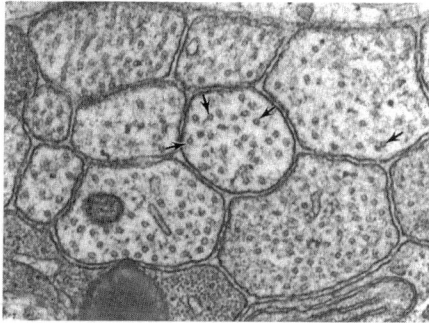

A: microfilaments
B: microtubules
C: intermediate filaments
D: actin filaments
E: cytokeratin filaments

Learning Response B: Correct. Microtubules are important constituents of the cytoskeleton and have a variety of functions within cells. Typically, they consist of 25 nm diameter tubes lined by alpha and beta tubulin molecules. Actin filaments or microfilaments would be approximately a fifth of the diameter of microtubules. Cytokeratin filaments are a class of intermediate filaments and would be intermediate in size between microtubules and microfilaments. Intermediate filaments and microfilaments are not hollow structures.

47.   SUBJECT AREA: Cytology
QUESTION: Identify the structures labeled by the arrows in the figure below.

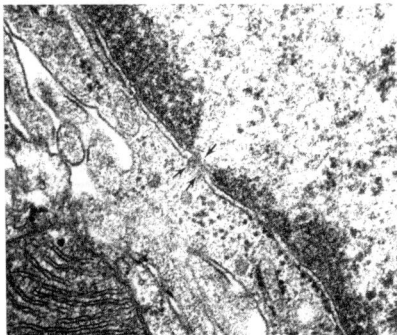

A: nuclear envelope
B: fibrous lamina
C: nuclear pores
D: euchromatin
E: perinuclear cisterna

Learning Response C: Correct. Nuclear pores allow the passage of material to and from the cytoplasm. Proteins synthesized in the cytoplasm are transported to the nucleus. Ribonucleoprotein particles assembled in the nucleus exit through the nuclear pores, as does messenger RNA.

48.   SUBJECT AREA: Cytology
QUESTION: What stage of mitosis is depicted in the figure below?

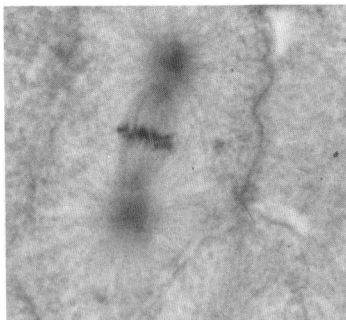

A: anaphase
B: metaphase

C: telophase
D: prophase
E: interphase

Learning Response B: Correct. The nuclear envelope is not visible.
Condensed chromosomes aligned along an equatorial plate in the center of
the mitotic spindle are characteristic of mitotic metaphase.

---

49.   SUBJECT AREA: Cytology
           QUESTION: What is the function of the cell depicted in the figure
           below?

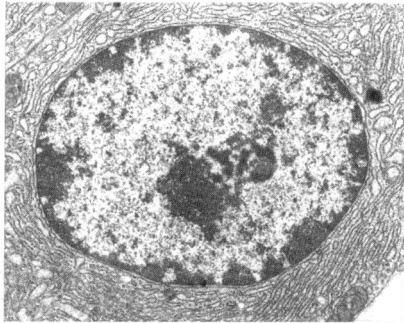

A: synthesis and secretion of proteins
B: synthesis and secretion of steroid hormones
C: cholesterol biosynthesis
D: phagocytosis
E: lipid storage

Learning Response A: Correct. The layers of rough endoplasmic reticulum
and a prominent nucleolus indicate that this cell makes proteins, many of
which would be secreted. Cells involved in lipid metabolism and
steroidogenesis would have smooth endoplasmic reticulum, large numbers of
mitochondria and lipid droplets.

50. SUBJECT AREA: Cytology

QUESTION: Identify the predominant cytoplasmic structure in the figure below.

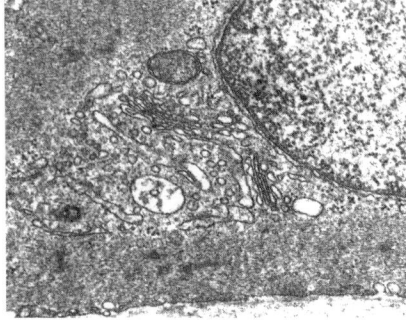

A: lipid droplets
B: smooth endoplasmic reticulum
C: lysosomes
D: rough endoplasmic reticulum
E: Golgi complex

Learning Response E: Correct. The flattened cisternae and transport vesicles associated with the cis face provide clues that this is the Golgi complex. The stacks of membrane that constitute the Golgi are not physically connected with each other, and vesicles shuttle from one level to the next.

51. SUBJECT AREA: Epithelial Tissue

QUESTION: Identify the type of epithelium depicted in the figure below.

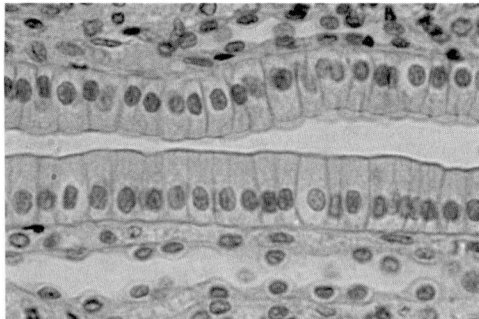

A: simple cuboidal

B: simple columnar
C: simple squamous
D: stratified columnar
E: stratified cuboidal

Learning Response B: Correct. Simple columnar cells are tall, rectangular cells with basal nuclei all at the same level. They usually have either absorptive or secretory functions, hence are found lining much of the digestive system and the larger ducts of glands.

52. Subject Area: Epithelial Tissue
Question The following are all primary functions of epithelial cells EXCEPT

A: calcium ion storage.
B: absorption.
C: contractility.
D: protection.
E: secretion.

Learning Response A: Correct. The principal functions of epithelial cells are absorption (gut), lining and covering of surfaces (skin), contractility (myoepithelial cells), exocrine and endocrine secretion and sensation (neuroepithelium).

53. Subject Area: Epithelial Tissue
Question: The lining of the respiratory system, the digestive tract, and the glands of the digestive tract is derived from which of the following embryonic germ layers?

A: ectoderm
B: endoderm
C: mesoderm

Learning Response B: Correct. The epithelium of the skin, mouth, nose and anus is derived from the ectoderm, the endothelial lining of blood vessels originates from mesoderm, and the lining of the respiratory system, the digestive tract and the glands of the digestive tract is derived from the endoderm.

54. SUBJECT AREA: Epithelial Tissue
QUESTION: The basal lamina, which separates and connects epithelial cells to connective tissue,

   A: consists of three layers: lamina densa, lamina lucida and lamina propria.
   B: is composed mainly of type V collagen.
   C: contains anchoring fibrils formed by type VII collagen which binds the basal lamina to adjacent collagen.
   D: contains a glycocalyx.
   E: contains tight junctions which anchor epithelial cells to the basal lamina.

Learning Response C: Correct. The basal lamina consists of the lamina rara and lamina densa and mainly is composed of type IV collagen, but also contains type VII collagen. Type VII collagen and bundles of microfibrils are part of the elastic elements of the superficial dermis.

55. SUBJECT AREA: Epithelial Tissue
QUESTION: Identify the tissue surrounding the luman in the figure below.

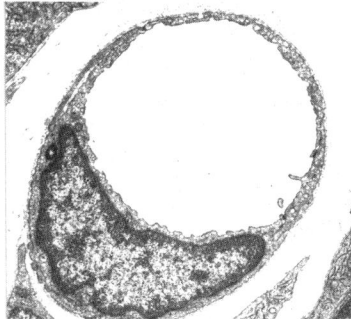

   A: simple columnar epithelium
   B: stratified squamous epithelium
   C: simple cuboidal epithelium
   D: simple squamous epithelium
   E: transitional epithelium

Learning Response D: Correct. The capillary is lined by endothelium or simple squamous epithelium, a single layer of flattened cells.

---

56. SUBJECT AREA: Epithelial Tissue
QUESTION: The microvilli shown in the figure below consist of

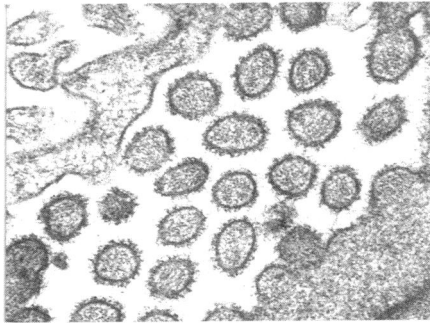

    A: myosin-containing filaments that are cross-linked to each other.
    B: strands of tropomyosin filaments that are cross-linked to each other.
    C: microtubules.
    D: actin-containing microfilaments that are cross-linked to each other and to the plasma membrane.
    E: tubular mitochondria aligned in a single row.

Learning Response D: Correct. Microvilli contain a cluster of 20-30 actin-containing microfilaments that are cross-linked to each other and to the surrounding plasma membrane by several different actin-binding proteins.

---

57. SUBJECT AREA: Epithelial Tissue
QUESTION: Pseudostratified epithelium can be found

    A: lining the respiratory tract.
    B: lining the digestive tract.
    C: covering the ovary and thyroid.
    D: lining the blood vessels.
    E: lining the urinary system.

Learning Response A: Correct. Pseudostratified epithelium consists of layers of cells with nuclei at different levels, but not all the cells reach the lumenal surface. This type of epithelium lines the nasal cavity, trachea and bronchi of the respiratory tract.

---

58. SUBJECT AREA: Epithelial Tissue
QUESTION: Basal bodies

> *A:* are electron-dense structures located at the apical pole just below the cell membrane of epithelial cells.
> *B:* form the base of all cilia.
> *C:* contain 9 sets of microtubule triplets arranged in a pinwheel fashion.
> *D:* are analogous to centrioles.
> *E:* contain all of the above characteristics.

Learning Response E: Correct. Each cilium has a basal body from which it is formed. The basal bodies act as a template to control the assembly of the axoneme subunits (9 + 2 arrangement of microtubules). Each of the 9 peripheral doublets shares 2-3 heterodimers. Adjacent doublets are linked to each other via protein bridges called nexins, and are linked to the central sheath by radial spokes. The central pair of tubules are separated from each other and are enclosed within a central sheath.

---

59. SUBJECT AREA: Epithelial Tissue
QUESTION: All of the following are characteristics of the basal lamina EXCEPT that

> *A:* it regulates exchanges of macromolecules between connective tissue and other tissues.
> *B:* it can be found between adjacent epithelial layers.
> *C:* the components of the basal lamina are secreted by epithelial, muscle, adipose and Schwann cells.
> *D:* it can only be seen with an electron microscope.
> *E:* it cannot facilitate cell-cell interactions.

Learning Response E: Correct. The basal lamina seems to contain information necessary for certain cell-cell interactions. An example of this is the reinnervation of denervated muscle cells.

---

60.   SUBJECT AREA: Epithelial Tissue
QUESTION: The main function of the structure labeled by the arrowheads in the figure below is to

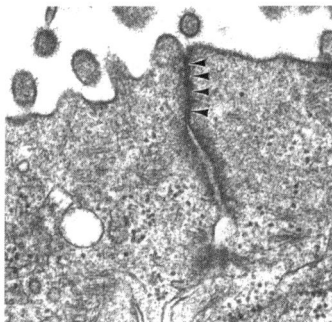

A: allow interchange of molecules with a molecular weight less than 1500 daltons between cells.
B: allow chemical communication between two epithelial cells.
C: form a tight seal that prevents the flow of material into the connective tissue between epithelial cells.
D: anchor the epithelium to the basal lamina.
E: provide rigidity to the apex of the cell.

Learning Response C: Correct. Zonula occludens, a belt consisting of tight junctions, forms a tight seal that prevents the flow of materials between epithelial cells. Tight or occluding junctions are the most apical of the components of the junctional complex in epithelial cells and are found in a number of other cell types, e.g., hepatocytes where they seal off the bile canaliculi.

61. SUBJECT AREA: Epithelial Tissue
QUESTION: The following are characteristics of epithelial tissue
EXCEPT that it

A: lacks blood vessels.
B: has a high regenerative capacity.
C: adheres to a basal lamina.
D: has little intercellular space.
E: lacks intermediate filaments in its cells.

Learning Response E: Correct. Ultrastructural and immunocytochemical studies reveal that intermediate filaments are present in almost all eukaryotic cells. In epithelial cells the intermediate filaments consist mainly of the protein keratin.

62. SUBJECT AREA: Epithelial Tissue
QUESTION: Exocrine glands

A: discharge secretory products via ducts.
B: discharge secretory products by diffusion directly
into the bloodstream.
C: secrete products only by constitutive mechanisms.
D: are only activated by genetic mechanisms.
E: secretes products known as hormones.

Learning Response A: Correct. Exocrine glands discharge their secretory products through ducts onto an epithelial surface. The activity of the gland depends on two types of regulated mechanisms: genetic and environmental controls from the nervous and endocrine systems.

63. SUBJECT AREA: Epithelial Tissue
QUESTION: Cells with absorptive properties will have an epithelial
lining

A: with cilia.
B: that consists of nonkeratinized stratified epithelium.
C: without a glycocalyx.

D: that is pseudostratified.

E: with a terminal web lying immediately beneath the lumenal surface.

Learning Response E: Correct. The cytoplasmic core of each microvillus contains actin microfilaments which insert into the terminal web. The terminal web is a specialization of the cytoskeleton lying immediately beneath the cell surface.

---

64. SUBJECT AREA: Epithelial Tissue

QUESTION: Epithelial cells of the proximal and distal renal tubules or the striated ducts of salivary glands

A: use a passive diffusion mechanism down a concentration gradient to transport sodium ions across the basal membrane of the cell.

B: are not all polarized cells.

C: maintain an osmotic balance by allowing an equimolar amount of Br^- and water into the cell along with Na^+.

D: have basal surfaces that are elaborately folded.

E: have none of the above characteristics.

Learning Response D: Correct. Within the folds of the basal surfaces are localized Mg^{2+}-activated Na^+/K^+ ATPase enzymes. Between the invaginations are vertically oriented mitochondria that supply the energy (ATP) for the active extrusions of Na^+ from the base of the cell.

---

65. SUBJECT AREA: Epithelial Tissue

QUESTION: Pinocytotic vesicles

A: have been shown to pass through a cell within 2-3 minutes.

B: appear in cells that have large quantities of rough endoplasmic reticulum and lysosomes.

C: flow through the cell in only one direction: apical to basal.

D: are formed from the rough endoplasmic reticulum of the cell.

E: permit the flow of hormones across the plasma membrane.

Learning Response A: Correct. Studies using electron-dense colloidal particles show that pinocytotic vesicles flow either from apical to basal locations or from basal to apical locations within the cell surfaces, but pass through the cells within 2-3 minutes. Pinocytotic vesicles are abundantly formed on plasmalemma surfaces of cells containing few organelles to allow the transport of macromolecules across the plasma membrane.

66.   SUBJECT AREA: Epithelial Tissue

QUESTION: The figure below is an electron micrograph of a cell actively involved in

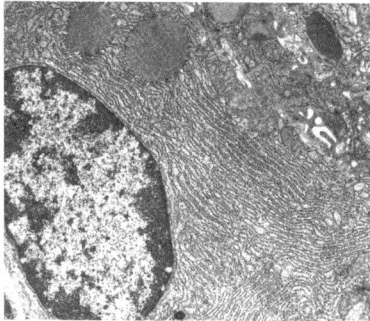

A: hormonal synthesis and storage.
B: protein synthesis and storage.
C: gamete formation.
D: absorption.
E: transporting chemical messages via synapses.

Learning Response B: Correct. The large amount of rough endoplasmic reticulum indicates that this cell is actively synthesizing protein. The accumulation of protein rich, membrane bound granules suggests that the cell is storing the product until it is triggered to release its product.

67.   SUBJECT AREA: Epithelial Tissue

QUESTION: Which one of the following sequences of events is in the correct order for protein synthesis, segregations and secretion to occur?

A: messenger RNA (mRNA), rough endoplasmic reticulum (RER), cis Golgi face, trans Golgi face, membrane bound secretory granules, exocytosis

B: RER, mRNA, cis Golgi face, trans Golgi face, membrane bound secretory granules, exocytosis

C: mRNA, RER, membrane bound secretory granules, trans Golgi face, cis Golgi face, exocytosis

D: RER, mRNA, membrane bound secretory granules, trans Golgi face, cis Golgi face, exocytosis

E: mRNA, RER, trans Golgi face, cis Golgi face, membrane bound secretory granules, exocytosis

Learning Response A: Correct. Some cells synthesize, segregate and secrete proteins without storing them (a process known as constitutive secretion, as opposed to regulated secretion in which the products are stored in the cytoplasm and secreted in response to a specific signal). In cells undergoing regulated secretion, proteins are synthesized from mRNA in the RER and transferred to the cis face of the Golgi complex. Within the Golgi complex, the proteins are sorted, and are further modified, if necessary. Membrane bound secretory granules bud off from the trans cisterna of the Golgi and are transported to the cell surface where their content is released by exocytosis.

68. SUBJECT AREA: Epithelial Tissue

QUESTION: The mechanism by which cells secrete a compound that acts upon neighboring target cells is called

A: paracrine secretion.

B: neurocrine secretion.

C: endocrine secretion.

D: exocrine secretion.

E: by none of the above choices.

Learning Response A: Correct. Cells that secrete via a paracrine method produce a substance that diffuses into the surrounding extracellular matrix and then acts upon neighboring target cells.

69. SUBJECT AREA: Epithelial Tissue
QUESTION: Three important structures found in the figure below that indicate this is a steroid-producing cell are

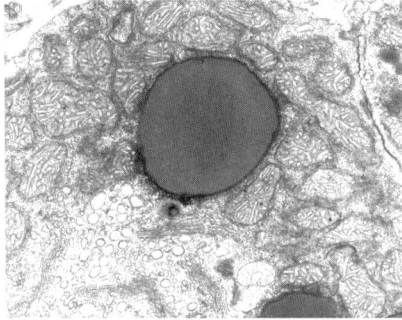

A: ribosomes, smooth endoplasmic reticulum (SER) and Golgi complex.
B: lipid, lysosomes and mitochondria.
C: SER, mitochondria and lipid.
D: lysosomes, mitochondria and Golgi complex.
E: ribosomes, mitochondria and Golgi complex.

Learning Response C: Correct. The cytoplasm of steroid-secreting cells is rich in SER which contains the necessary enzymes to synthesize cholesterol. Mitochondria not only contain the necessary enzymatic components to cleave cholesterol side chains and produce pregnenolone, but also participate in subsequent reactions that result in steroid hormones. An abundance of lipid droplets is usually, but not always, found in steroid-secreting cells.

70. SUBJECT AREA: Epithelial Tissue
QUESTION: Myoepithelial cells

A: are connected to each other by desmosomes and tight junctions.
B: contain tropomyosin and myosin confirming their epithelial origin.
C: are located between the basal lamina and the basal surface of secretory or ductal cells.
D: can be found in skeletal muscle.
E: contain myofibrils.

Learning Response C: Correct. Myoepithelial cells are located between the basal lamina and the basal pole of secretory or ductal cells. They are connected to each other by desmosomes and gap junctions. Their cytoplasm contains actin, tropomyosin and myosin (characteristic of muscle cells), and intermediate filaments belonging to the cytokeratin family (characteristic of epithelial origin). Contraction of myoepithelial cells helps to extrude secretory products from the gland and/or out the ducts.

---

71. SUBJECT AREA: Epithelial Tissue

QUESTION: All of the following are morphologic characteristics of cells of the diffuse neuroendocrine system EXCEPT

    A: vesicles with a dense core.

    B: vesicles concentrated at the basal portion of the cell.

    C: immunocytochemical identification of a biogenic amine or polypeptide hormone.

    D: will result in a decrease in hormonal secretion when malignancy occurs (apudomas).

    E: scattered throughout an epithelium, but not necessarily in contact with the lumenal surface.

Learning Response D: Correct. DNES cells can be identified for a specific amine and localized using immunocytochemical methods. They are polypeptide-secreting cells with dense core granules about 100-400 nm in diameter that are located at the basal pole of the cell. Cells producing peptides or amines have a greater amount of rough endoplasmic reticulum than smooth endoplasmic reticulum. A cell which contains a large amount of smooth endoplasmic reticulum is most likely producing steroid hormones, not peptide hormones.

---

72. SUBJECT AREA: Epithelial Tissue

QUESTION: In stratified squamous epithelium,

    A: proliferation occurs throughout the tissue.

    B: the basal layer of cells is flattened and enucleated.

    C: a thick layer of keratin is a constant feature.

    D: papillation brings basal cells closer to their source of nutrition.

    E: cells are attached to the basal lamina by half

desmosomes (hemidesmosomes).

Learning Response E: Correct. Proliferation of stratified squamous epithelium occurs in the basal layer of cells which are rounded and nucleated. Keratin is absent on moist membranes, and papillation brings the cells in the outer layers closer to nutrients brought by capillaries in the underlying connective tissue. The epithelium is anchored to the basal lamina by hemidesmosomes.

73. SUBJECT AREA: Epithelial Tissue
QUESTION: A feature which is characteristic of all epithelial tissue is

> *A:* cell surface modification, such as cilia or microvilli.
> *B:* association with the basal lamina.
> *C:* keratinization.
> *D:* the presence of goblet cells.
> *E:* vascularization.

Learning Response B: Correct. All of the different types of epithelial tissues rest on a basal lamina. Not all epithelia have surface modifications, keratin or goblet cells, and none have blood vessels.

74. SUBJECT AREA: Epithelial Tissue
QUESTION: Transitional epithelium

> *A:* represents a "transitional tissue" between stratified squamous and stratified cuboidal epithelium.
> *B:* can exhibit binucleate cells in its uppermost layer.
> *C:* often has stereocilia as a surface modification.
> *D:* is usually one cell layer thick.
> *E:* is often associated with the respiratory tract.

Learning Response B: Correct. Transitional epithelium is found in the urinary tract and can change the shape of the surface cells from a dome shape to a flattened shape depending on the degree of distention of the organ. Often the surface cells have more than one nucleus.

---

75. SUBJECT AREA: Epithelial Tissue

QUESTION: Which of the following *cannot* be considered a member of the diffuse neuroendocrine system (DNES)?

A: carotid bodies (intercarotid paraganglia)
B: thyroid parafollicular cells
C: gastrin-secreting cells in the stomach
D: pulmonary neuroepithelial cells
E: adrenal medullary cells

Learning Response E: Correct. Adrenomedullary cells are actually modified postganglionic sympathetic neurons. DNES cells are not confined to the digestive system. It is important to note that the presence of an ectopic hormone-producing cell in biopsy is indicative of a cell of DNES origin and can be found almost anywhere in the body.

---

76. SUBJECT AREA: Epithelial Tissue

QUESTION: All of the following statements about communicating (gap) junctions are true EXCEPT that they

A: are regions of low electrical resistance between cells.
B: exhibit a narrow intercellular space approximately 2-4 nm in width.
C: allow proteins (5,000-10,000 daltons molecular weight) to pass from one cell to the next.
D: contain structures called connexons which form a bridge between the cells.
E: can be found in smooth muscle cells in which they allow the cells to function as a physiological syncytium.

Learning Response C: Correct. Ions are readily passed through the connexons of communicating junctions while low molecular weight proteins are restricted.

---

77. SUBJECT AREA: Epithelial Tissue
QUESTION: Identify the type of cell depicted in the figure below.

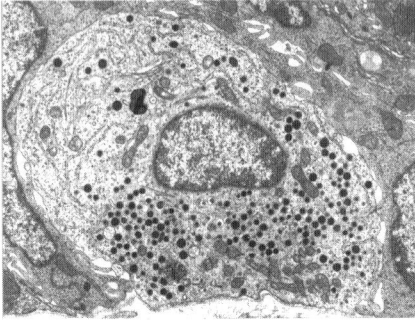

A: goblet cell
B: cell of the diffuse neuroendocrine system
C: absorptive epithelial cell
D: steroid-secreting cell
E: pancreatic acinar cell

Learning Response B: Correct. The basal location of dense core granules is the major clue in the identification of this type of cell.

---

78. SUBJECT AREA: Epithelial Tissue
QUESTION: The type of cell-cell junction illustrated in the figure below and labeled by a number 2 is a

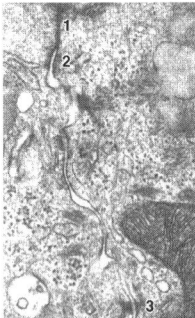

A: spot desmosome.
B: occluding junction.
C: band desmosome.
D: communicating junction.
E: hemidesmosome.

Learning Response C: Correct. Thickening of the cytoplasmic surface of the plasma membrane, insertion of microfilaments into the thickened plasma membrane and the wide intercellular space are typical features of band desmosomes. The numbers 1 and 3 refer to occluding junction and spot desmosome, respectively. Hemidesmosomes would be located at the base of the cell adjacent to the basement membrane, not along the lateral surface. Communicating junctions exhibit a very narrow gap between the two adjacent cells.

79. SUBJECT AREA: Connective Tissue
QUESTION: In reference to connective tissues,

    A: there is a higher concentration of collagen fibers in loose connective tissue (CT) than in dense CT.
    B: macrophages are generally incapable of movement since they lack an actin cytoskeleton.
    C: mast cell granules can contain the small proteoglycan, hyaluronic acid.
    D: cell surface proteoglycans (PG) such as heparan sulfate PG can function in cell adhesion.
    E: elastic fibers are components of the basal lamina.

Learning Response D: Correct. In addition to their role as components of the extracellular matrix (ECM), proteoglycans may also be located at the surface of cells and, as such, can function in cell adhesion. By definition, dense connective tissue has more collagen fibrils and fewer cells than loose connective tissue. Macrophages are mobile, and mast cells contain heparin as their proteoglycan; hyaluronic acid is a glycosaminoglycan in the ECM.

80. SUBJECT AREA: Connective Tissue
QUESTION: The basal lamina or basement membrane

A: contains laminin which, through its association with entactin (nidogen), can bind to type IV collagen.
B: allows for the diffusion of nutrients to epithelial cells.
C: is present around muscle cells.
D: has an active role in such processes as cell differentiation and cell spreading.
E: can be characterized by all of the above features.

Learning Response E: Correct. The basal lamina is an important structure that provides contact and communication between epithelial cells or muscle cells or nerve cells and the extracellular matrix.

81. SUBJECT AREA: Connective Tissue
QUESTION: All of the following are features of plasma cells EXCEPT

A: a heterochromatic nucleus.
B: they are derived from blood basophils.
C: the presence of a Golgi complex.
D: a prominent rough endoplasmic reticulum.
E: a prominent nucleolus.

Learning Response B: Correct. Plasma cells represent the terminal stage of differentiation of B lymphocytes activated by the presence of antigen. These cells contain all of the organelles consistent with the constitutive synthesis and secretion of antibody proteins.

82. SUBJECT AREA: Connective Tissue
QUESTION: As part of a summer research project, you have isolated mutant fibroblasts which produce glycoproteins with deleted R-G-D (arg-gly-asp) amino acid sequences. Which event(s) would be affected by this deletion?

A: Binding of α-actinin to actin microfilaments
B: Binding of fibronectin to type III collagen
C: Binding of laminin to type IV collagen
D: Binding of fibronectin to integrins

E: Binding of integrins to cytoskeletal proteins

Learning Response D: Correct. The extracellular glycoprotein fibronectin has a specific sequence of amino acids that allows it to bind to integrins, integral membrane proteins at the surface of epithelial cells. This permits communication between intracellular and extracellular events.

---

83. SUBJECT AREA: Connective Tissue
QUESTION: In studying the lamina densa in detail, one would observe that it

A: contains high levels of type I collagen.
B: serves as a termination point of anchoring fibrils containing type IV collagen.
C: is particularly abundant around mesenchymal cells.
D: is readily seen at the light microscope level when stained with hematoxylin and eosin.
E: has heparan sulfate proteoglycan associated with it.

Learning Response E: Correct. The lamina densa can only be visualized with the electron microscope and contains a high concentration of heparan sulfate proteoglycan. Anchoring fibrils are composed of type VII collagen and do terminate in the lamina densa. Type IV collagen is located in the basal lamina.

---

84. SUBJECT AREA: Connective Tissue
QUESTION: Hormones can

A: inhibit the synthesis of collagen.
B: have a detrimental effect on wound healing.
C: suppress the actions of the cells of the immune system in connective tissue.
D: produce an accumulation of glycosaminoglycans in connective tissue.
E: have all of the above effects.

Learning Response E: Correct. A number of different hormones affect the metabolic activity and function of the components of connective tissue. Cortisol from the adrenal cortex inhibits collagen fibrillogenesis, and ACTH can reduce the efficiency of wound healing. Both hormones can suppress lymphocytic and plasmacytic activities. Hypothyroidism results in the accumulation of glycosaminoglycans in connective tissue.

---

85. SUBJECT AREA: Connective Tissue

QUESTION: Which of the following statements is correct regarding the biosynthesis and assembly of the different extracellular matrix constituents?

A: Mutations altering the primary structure of the collagen molecule can contribute to deficiencies in collagen assembly.

B: Cleavage of extension peptides is essential for proper assembly of type IV collagen into fibers.

C: Type II and type IX collagens represent the major collagens in tendons.

D: Procollagen peptidase is active in the endoplasmic reticulum.

E: Type I collagen assembles into fibrils which are found in secretory vesicles.

Learning Response A: Correct. Type IV collagen does not form fibrils; types I and V are located in tendons. Type II and type IX collagens are found in cartilage. In extracellular matrix, procollagen peptidase cleaves the nonhelical regions of procollagen allowing it to form tropocollagen. Fibril assembly of type I collagen occurs extracellularly.

---

86. SUBJECT AREA: Connective Tissue

QUESTION: Regions in which dense regular connective tissue would be located include

A: lamina propria of the duodenum.

B: the skin.

C: organ capsules.

D: the superficial fascia.

E: ligaments and tendons.

Learning Response E: Correct. The primary location of dense regular connective tissue would be in tendons and ligaments. Dense irregular tissue is located in the dermis of the skin and in the capsules of organs such as the kidney. Loose connective tissue is found in the lamina propria of the gastrointestinal tract and in the superficial fascia.

87. SUBJECT AREA: Connective Tissue
QUESTION: The principal amino acids in collagen include all of the following EXCEPT

    A: hydroxylysine.
    B: tryptophan.
    C: hydroxyproline.
    D: glycine.
    E: proline.

Learning Response B: Correct. Collagen is 10% hydroxyproline, 12% proline and 33.5% glycine. Hydroxyproline and hydroxylysine are unique to collagen, and the content of tryptophan in collagen is uninteresting.

88. SUBJECT AREA: Connective Tissue
QUESTION: Mast cells store all of the following substances in membrane bound secretory granules EXCEPT

    A: histamine.
    B: chondroitin sulfate.
    C: leukotriene.
    D: heparin.
    E: proteases.

Learning Response C: Correct. Leukotriene, formerly known as slow reactive substance of anaphylaxis, is synthesized and secreted on demand and not stored in the cytoplasmic granules prior to release.

89. SUBJECT AREA: Connective Tissue

QUESTION: In the synthesis and assembly of collagen fibrils, vitamin C acts as a

A: component of the procollagen molecule.

B: cofactor needed for the assembly of alpha chains in the extracellular space.

C: cofactor of peptidyl proline hydroxylase.

D: cofactor for conversion of lysine to hydroxylysine.

E: crosslinking agent allowing for the formation of fibers from fibrils.

Learning Response C: Correct. Vitamin C acts as a cofactor for the conversion of proline to hydroxyproline. Deficiencies in this vitamin produce a condition called scurvy characterized by a degeneration of connective tissue. Resultant defective fibrillogenesis occurs especially in areas of high collagen turnover such as the periodontal ligaments which hold teeth in their sockets.

90. SUBJECT AREA: Connective Tissue

QUESTION: As a result of a bee sting, a person comes to a physician with general swelling in the area of the sting, difficulty in breathing and a bluish complexion. The physician decides that the person has had an immediate hypersensitivity reaction. What would you expect to see in the connective tissue of this person upon biopsy (or upon autopsy if immediate treatment were neglected)?

A: proliferation of monocytes

B: degranulation of mast cells

C: increased number of plasma cells

D: localized accumulation of T lymphocytes

E: proliferation of fibroblasts in the area of the sting

Learning Response B: Correct. Mast cells sensitized by a previous immunologic reaction to bee venom are capable of binding immunoglobulin E (IgE) at their surface. Subsequent contact with the antigen by IgE produces a rapid degranulation of mast cells and the release of the contents of the granules into the extracellular matrix. Enhanced pharmacological effects of the substances secreted by these mast cells can endanger the health of the sensitized individual.

---

91. SUBJECT AREA: Connective Tissue
QUESTION: Loose or areolar connective tissue

        A: contains mostly reticular fibers.
        B: can be found at the insertion of skeletal muscle into tendon.
        C: is located in the anterior cruciate ligament of the knee joint.
        D: can exhibit accumulations of lymphocytes in response to localized immune reactions.
        E: characteristically lacks capillaries.

Learning Response D: Correct. As part of the defense function of connective tissue, lymphocytes present in loose connective tissue can respond to antigenic stimulation. Tendons and ligaments are examples of dense connective tissue. Relatively few reticular fibers are found in loose connective tissue.

---

92. SUBJECT AREA: Connective Tissue
QUESTION: Elastic fibers are common in

        A: the aorta.
        B: alveoli.
        C: the dermis.
        D: the hypodermis.
        E: all of the above areas.

Learning Response E: Correct. Elastic fibers are widely distributed; however, in examining histological sections, the ubiquity of these structures can only be appreciated by special stains which demonstrate elastic fibers.

---

93. SUBJECT AREA: Connective Tissue
QUESTION: In connective tissue,

A: elastic fibers and reticular fibers can be demonstrated by the same histological stain.

B: neutrophils and eosinophils are present, having migrated from blood.

C: mast cells in the mucosal and connective tissues represent homogeneous populations.

D: fibroblasts are an undifferentiated cell type.

E: macrophages are readily visible in the vicinity of blood vessels in routinely stained (H & E) histological sections.

Learning Response B: Correct. In defending the body from infections, neutrophils and eosinophils are mobilized from blood and enter connective tissues where they function to neutralize bacteria and other microorganisms. Mast cell populations are heterogeneous; mucosal and connective tissue cells have different types of proteoglycan in their granules. Fibroblasts are mature cells which synthesize and secrete the components of the matrix. Macrophages are difficult to demonstrate in routinely stained sections and require special dyes. Lastly, reticular fibers can be stained with silver salts, and elastic fibers have no affinity for silver.

94.   SUBJECT AREA: Connective Tissue

QUESTION: All of the following are features of collagen fibrils EXCEPT that they

A: assemble while encased by the cytoplasm of fibroblasts.

B: may contain more than one type of collagen.

C: exhibit a 64-67 nm periodicity in electron micrographs.

D: contain amino acids which are hydroxylated in the rough endoplasmic reticulum.

E: are found in all three types of cartilage.

Learning Response A: Correct. Procollagen molecules are secreted into the extracellular matrix where peptidases remove nonhelical regions of the molecules transforming procollagen into tropocollagen which assembles into fibrils which are crosslinked into fibers.

95. SUBJECT AREA: Connective Tissue

   QUESTION: In the responses of connective tissue to an allergic reaction to pollen, all of the following events occur EXCEPT

   A: mast cells bind IgE antibodies at their surfaces.

   B: fibroblasts secrete more collagen and elastin to sequester pollen.

   C: eosinophils produce histaminase to modulate the activity of mast cells.

   D: mast cell granule release is mediated by the binding of pollen antigen to cell surface antibodies.

   E: increased vascular permeability results from the secretion of the products of mast cells.

Learning Response B: Correct. Fibroblasts do not function in fibrillogenesis in response to allergic reactions.

96. SUBJECT AREA: Connective Tissue

   QUESTION: Macrophages

   A: are normally multinucleated cells.

   B: synthesize and release immunoglobulins.

   C: are phagocytic cells derived from monocytes.

   D: have a prominent smooth endoplasmic reticulum.

   E: produce the extracellular matrix of loose connective tissue.

Learning Response C: Correct. Macrophages can function as phagocytic cells and as antigen presenting cells. They are derived from blood monocytes which migrate into connective tissue. Macrophages are normally singly nucleated and widely distributed in loose connective tissue. Multinucleated giant cells derived from macrophages can be located in connective tissue in certain pathological conditions. Plasma cells release immunoglobulins, and fibroblasts secrete matrix components.

97. SUBJECT AREA: Connective Tissue

QUESTION: In reference to the extracellular matrix (ECM) of loose connective tissue,

A: fibronectin and laminin are the principal ECM glycoproteins.

B: fibrillar forms of collagen are often associated with other, nonfibrillar, collagens.

C: its components can interact directly with proteins in epithelial cell membranes to anchor these cells to the underlying connective tissue.

D: crosslinking of desmosine and isodesmosine residues of elastin accounts for the protein's elasticity.

E: all of the above statements are correct.

Learning Response E: Correct. The ECM contains a wide variety of proteins and polysaccharides and exhibits a multiplicity of functions.

98. SUBJECT AREA: Connective Tissue

QUESTION: All of the following are characteristic of reticular fibers EXCEPT that they

A: are composed primarily of type III collagen.

B: are located in the connective tissue framework of lymph nodes and the spleen.

C: allow for changes in shape of several organs, e.g., spleen and liver.

D: are PAS-negative, reflecting a lack of associated glycoproteins.

E: can be linked by proteoglycans.

Learning Response D: Correct. Reticular fibers are PAS-positive because of their high content of glycoproteins.

99. SUBJECT AREA: Connective Tissue

QUESTION: Classify the type of connective tissue (CT) found in the figure below.

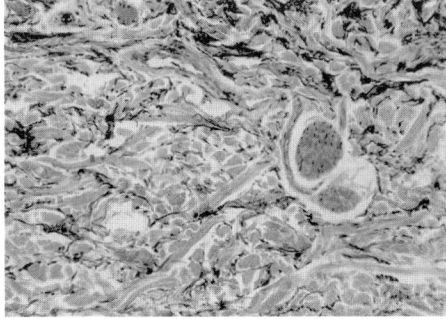

A: loose or areolar CT
B: dense irregular CT
C: reticular CT
D: elastic CT
E: mucous CT

Learning Response B: Correct. The presence of densely packed collagen fibers and the sparsity of cells are characteristic of dense CT. In this image, the collagen fibers are not arranged in a regular pattern such as those found in tendons, and therefore, the tissue is classified as dense irregular CT. The darkly stained structures are elastic fibers.

100. SUBJECT AREA: Connective Tissue

QUESTION: Identify the type of connective tissue fibers in the figure below.

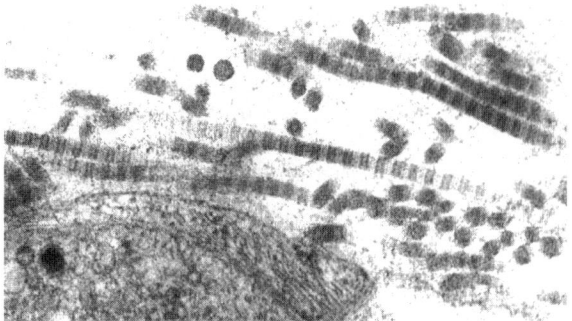

A: collagen
B: elastic
C: reticular
D: choices A and C above
E: choices B and C above

Learning Response D: Correct. Type I and type III collagen can form fibers. However, type III fibers are smaller in diameter than type I fibers. Unfortunately, there is no basis for this comparison in the electron micrograph in the figure.

---

101. SUBJECT AREA: Connective Tissue
QUESTION: What is the function of the type of cell depicted in the figure below?

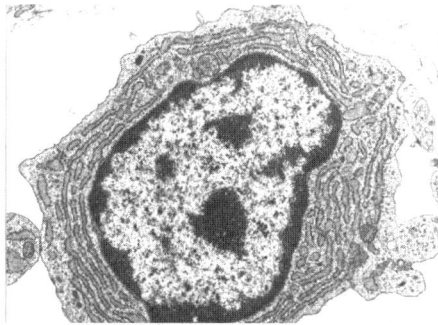

A: fibrillogenesis
B: phagocytosis
C: immunoglobulin secretion
D: histamine secretion
E: histaminase secretion

Learning Response C: Correct. The cell is a plasma cell which functions in immune reactions by synthesizing and secreting immunoglobulin molecules. Fibroblasts are responsible for the production of proteins which form fibers. Macrophages are active in phagocytosis; mast cells release histamine, and eosinophils produce histaminase which counteracts the effects of histamine.

102. SUBJECT AREA: Connective Tissue
QUESTION: Identify the nucleated cell shown in the figure below.

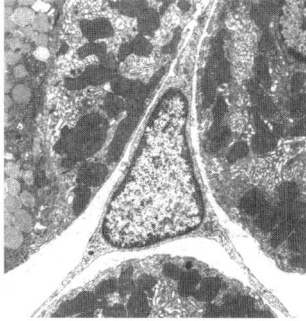

A: quiescent fibroblast
B: active macrophage
C: degranulated mast cell
D: activated lymphocyte
E: migrating eosinophil

Learning Response A: Correct. The stellate shape, central nucleus and attenuated cytoplasm indicate that the cell is a fibroblast. The absence of large amounts of rough endoplasmic reticulum suggests that the fibroblast may be inactive. An inactive or quiescent fibroblast can be called a fibrocyte.

103. SUBJECT AREA: Connective Tissue
QUESTION: The type of cell illustrated in the figure below functions in

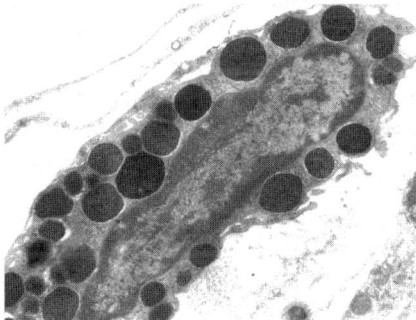

A: allergic reactions.

B: secretion of substances which increase vascular permeability.

C: secretion of substances which attract eosinophils.

D: secretion of heparin, an anticoagulant.

E: all of the above activities.

Learning Response E: Correct. Mast cells exhibit a multiplicity of important functions and are widely distributed in connective tissue.

---

104. SUBJECT AREA: Connective Tissue

QUESTION: The increase in the amount of fat stored in the body later in life is the result of

A: an increase in numbers of unilocular adipocytes.

B: a change in the amount of lipid stored by unilocular adipocytes.

C: changes in both size and numbers of unilocular adipocytes.

D: an increase in the amount of multilocular adipose tissue.

E: a change in the amount of lipid stored by multilocular adipocytes.

Learning Response B: Correct. The number of unilocular adipocytes can increase during a brief period of postnatal life, but after that the cells do not change appreciably in numbers. The cells can, however, accumulate more lipid during life. Multilocular fat (brown fat) is found primarily in the human embryo and in newborn infants. It is reduced in amount in adults.

---

105. SUBJECT AREA: Connective Tissue

QUESTION: A mutant in the adipocyte gene that encodes lipoprotein lipase, an enzyme which is transferred to the cell membrane of capillaries in adipose tissue, would most likely result in

A: the inability of capillaries to hydrolyze chylomicrons and very low density lipoproteins (VLDL).

> *B:* a rapid increase in the amount of lipid stored
> in adipocytes.
> *C:* no decrease in the amount of lipid stored
> in adipocytes.
> *D:* a decrease in the numbers of chylomicrons in
> the blood stream.
> *E:* the rapid accumulation of triglycerides
> in adipocytes.

Learning Response A: Correct. Lipoprotein lipase at the luminal surface of capillaries in adipose tissue breaks down chylomicrons and VLDL to triglycerides and cholesterol which are taken up by the adipocytes. The enzyme is transferred to the endothelial cells by adipocytes.

106. SUBJECT AREA: Connective Tissue
QUESTION: All of the following are features of multilocular adipose tissue EXCEPT that

> *A:* the cells contain several fat vacuoles.
> *B:* the cells contain large numbers of mitochondria.
> *C:* it is widely distributed throughout the body.
> *D:* it is abundant in hibernating animals.
> *E:* it has a large number of capillaries.

Learning Response C: Correct. Unlike white fat, brown fat is limited to the shoulder area and along the spine and rib cages of newborn infants. The amount of brown fat is greatly reduced in the adult.

107. SUBJECT AREA: Connective Tissue
QUESTION: The type of lipid stored in adipocytes is

> *A:* monoglycerides.
> *B:* diglycerides.
> *C:* triglycerides.
> *D:* phospholipid.
> *E:* fatty acids.

Learning Response C: Correct. Triglycerides which are esters of fatty acids and glycerol are stored in adipose tissue cells.

---

108. SUBJECT AREA: Connective Tissue

QUESTION: In routine hematoxylin and eosin stained histological sections, unilocular adipose cells have a signet ring shape with a rim of cytoplasm surrounding a clear space. This is the result of

A: the inability of the dyes to stain lipid molecules.

B: an artifact of fixation procedures.

C: breaks in the plasma membrane allowing leakage of lipid into the surrounding connective tissue.

D: the removal of the lipid by the organic solvents used to prepare the tissue.

E: less than optimum embedding in paraffin.

Learning Response D: Correct. Alcohol and xylol that are used in the dehydration and pre-embedding procedures dissolve the lipid from the cells. Fixation preserves cellular structure, and less than optimum embedding in paraffin would result in breaks or tears in the tissue.

---

109. SUBJECT AREA: Connective Tissue

QUESTION: The functions of adipose tissue include

A: thermal insulation of the body.

B: the absorption of compression shocks at the soles of the feet and palms of the hands.

C: the storage of caloric energy in the form of lipids.

D: the creation of monetary profits for the makers of exercise videotapes.

E: all of the above choices.

Learning Response E: Correct. Lipids in the form of triglycerides are stored in adipose tissue and can be mobilized quickly when needed. These lipids are poor conductors of heat and provide an insulation for the body. Fat pads in the palms and soles act as shock absorbers for the limbs. Adipose tissue also protects some of the soft organs, especially the kidneys, from injury or trauma.

110. SUBJECT AREA: Connective Tissue

QUESTION: The mobilization of stored lipids from adipocytes involves all of the following EXCEPT

A: the release of fatty acids and glycerol into the blood stream.

B: the influence of growth hormone, insulin and other hormones in the process.

C: increased synthesis of lipoprotein lipase.

D: the action of norepinephrine on the activation of triglyceride lipase.

E: the transport of insoluble fatty acids bound to serum albumin to other tissues of the body.

Learning Response C: Correct. Lipoprotein lipase is involved in the uptake of serum lipids from the blood stream to the capillaries and finally to the adipocytes.

111. SUBJECT AREA: Connective Tissue

QUESTION: Which of the following statements about adipose tissue is NOT correct?

A: Adipose cells are derived from lipoblasts which develop from mesenchymal cells.

B: In contrast to the lipid droplets stored in unilocular adipocytes, the lipid in multilocular cells is bound by a cell membrane.

C: Unilocular adipose cells can develop into benign tumors known as lipomas.

D: Both brown and white fat are highly vascular tissues.

E: Reticular fibers form part of the stroma that holds the adipocytes together.

Learning Response B: Correct. Both white and brown fat cells store lipid droplets which are not bound by cell membrane. Adipose tissue has numerous capillaries, can generate tumors and contains reticular fibers as the stromal framework. Adipose tissue is derived from mesenchyme.

112. SUBJECT AREA: Connective Tissue

QUESTION: In the figure below, identify the specialized type of connective tissue (CT).

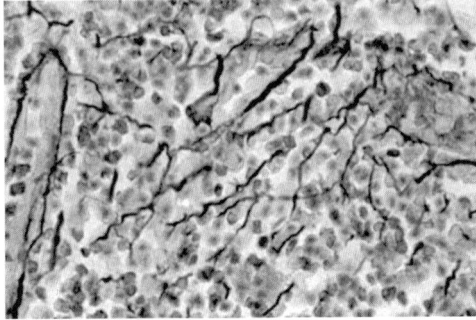

A: loose or areolar CT
B: elastic CT
C: dense CT
D: reticular CT
E: adipose CT

Learning Response D: Correct. The short, branched reticular fibers constitute the stroma of the organs of the lymphoid system. There the network of reticular fibers forms a special type of CT, reticular CT.

113. SUBJECT AREA: Connective Tissue

QUESTION: The cells in the figure below would most likely be located in which of the following regions of a one month old child?

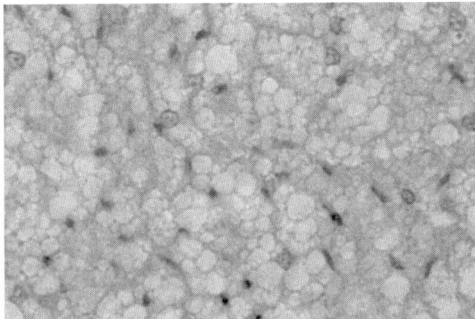

> A: brain
> B: gluteal region
> C: neck and abdominal regions
> D: upper limbs
> E: lower limbs

Learning Response C: Correct. Multilocular adipose tissue constitutes 2–5% of a newborn's body weight and is concentrated in the lateral aspects of the neck and upper abdominal regions. There is a mixture of white and brown fat in the shoulder area, but the other choices are devoid of multilocular fat.

114. SUBJECT AREA: Blood and Myeloid Tissue
QUESTION: Eosinophils

> A: have a diameter between 12 μm and 15 μm in blood smears.
> B: are found throughout the respiratory and gastrointestinal tracts.
> C: are observed in chronic inflammatory reactions.
> D: are produced in the bone marrow.
> E: exhibit all of the above features.

Learning Response E: Correct. Eosinophils are widely distributed in connective tissue having migrated there from the peripheral blood stream. They have a number of functions including the destruction of parasites such as schistosomes.

115. SUBJECT AREA: Blood and Myeloid Tissue
QUESTION: Erythrocytes

> A: normally enter the blood stream containing a single, pyknotic nucleus.
> B: become swollen when exposed to hypertonic solution.
> C: have a membrane skeleton that determines the shape of the cells.
> D: are destroyed in the liver, bone marrow and kidneys.

E: have a functional life span of less than 60 days.

Learning Response C: Correct. The biconcave shape of erythrocytes is determined by a complex membrane skeleton that includes the protein spectrin. Normally, red blood cells enter the circulation as reticulocytes which lack a nucleus. Erythrocytes have a life span of approximately 120 days. Nonfunctional red cells are removed by macrophages in the spleen and bone marrow. Exposure to hypertonic solutions will shrink red blood cells.

---

116. SUBJECT AREA: Blood and Myeloid Tissue
QUESTION: B lymphocytes can

> *A:* ingest pathogenic organisms.
> *B:* differentiate into plasma cells during immune responses.
> *C:* differentiate into macrophages as a result of tissue damage.
> *D:* secrete histamine, heparin and leukotriene C.
> *E:* remove effete erythrocytes from the peripheral blood stream.

Learning Response B: Correct. In response to antigenic stimulation and interactions with T lymphocytes and interleukins, B lymphocytes differentiate into plasma cells which secrete large amounts of immunoglobulins.

---

117. SUBJECT AREA: Blood and Myeloid Tissue
QUESTION: Platelets

> *A:* contain serotonin which is stored in granules.
> *B:* may become adherent when exposed to collagen.
> *C:* lack nuclei but contain actin and microtubules.
> *D:* function in clot retraction as well as clot formation.
> *E:* exhibit all of the above features.

Learning Response E: Correct. Platelets or thrombocytes are important in clotting mechanisms and contain a number of different types of granules and cytoskeletal proteins.

118. SUBJECT AREA: Blood and Myeloid Tissue
QUESTION: Serum

A: is synonymous with the term blood plasma.
B: contains plasma and red and white blood cells.
C: forms the buffy coat in the hematocrit tube.
D: is identical to plasma minus the clotting factors.
E: forms the interstitial fluid in loose connective tissue.

Learning Response D: Correct. Plasma is the fluid component of blood; serum is plasma without the clotting factors. The buffy coat in the hematocrit tube consists of leukocytes. Clinically it often useful to stain the buffy coat to look for causative organisms in cases of suspected sepsis.

119. SUBJECT AREA: Blood and Myeloid Tissue
QUESTION: The estimation of packed erythrocyte volume per unit volume of blood can be obtained by the centrifugation of blood and is known as the

A: sedimentation rate.
B: hematocrit.
C: hemoglobin volume.
D: buffy coat.
E: complete blood count or CBC.

Learning Response B: Correct. The hematocrit is the estimation of the volume of erythrocytes following centrifugation of blood treated with anticoagulants. The normal value is between 35-50% in adults.

120. SUBJECT AREA: Blood and Myeloid Tissue
QUESTION: All of the following are considered to be plasma proteins EXCEPT

A: immunoglobulins.
B: albumin.
C: fibrinogen.

D: erythropoietin.
E: alpha globulins.

Learning Response D: Correct. Erythropoietin is a hormone produced by the interstitial cells of the kidney and functions in the stimulation of red blood cell formation. It is not considered to be one of the plasma proteins.

121. SUBJECT AREA: Blood and Myeloid Tissue
QUESTION: The formed elements of blood include

A: platelets.
B: leukocytes.
C: plasma proteins.
D: choices A and B above.
E: choices A, B and C above.

Learning Response D: Correct. Plasma proteins are not considered to be part of the formed blood elements which include cells and parts of cells (platelets).

122. SUBJECT AREA: Blood and Myeloid Tissue
QUESTION: Hemoglobin exhibits all of the following EXCEPT that it

A: is the oxygen and carbon dioxide binding protein of erythrocytes.
B: normally is synthesized on polyribosomes in mature cells.
C: is one of several proteins found in the cytoplasm of mature cells.
D: can form a complex with carbon monoxide reducing its functional ability.
E: can have substitutions in one amino acid resulting in pathological changes in the cells.

Learning Response B: Correct. Hemoglobin synthesis occurs in the developmental stages of erythrocytes. Mature cells lack mitochondria and polyribosomes and, thus, do not synthesize proteins.

123. SUBJECT AREA: Blood and Myeloid Tissue
QUESTION: Eosinophils have all of the following features EXCEPT that they

A: are binucleate.
B: have ovoid, membrane bound granules which contain hydrolytic enzymes.
C: increase in the circulation in response to parasitic infestations.
D: are attracted by substances secreted by mast cells and basophils.
E: produce substances that deactivate vasoactive materials.

Learning Response A: Correct. Eosinophils contain a single, bilobed nucleus. Eosinophilic granules contain major basic protein which imparts an intense eosinophilic stain to the cells and may also function in the killing of parasites.

124. SUBJECT AREA: Blood and Myeloid Tissue
QUESTION: White blood cells or leukocytes

A: can be classified as granulocytes or agranulocytes.
B: can perform some of their functions outside the circulatory system.
C: known as monocytes are precursors of the cells of the mononuclear phagocytic system.
D: known as basophils have granules which contain heparin and histamine.
E: exhibit all of the above characteristics.

Learning Response E: Correct. The granulocytic (neutrophils, eosinophils and basophils) and agranulocytic (lymphocytes and monocytes) classes of leukocytes perform a variety of functions and are not restricted to the peripheral blood stream.

125. SUBJECT AREA: Blood and Myeloid Tissue
QUESTION: All of the following are components of the azurophilic granules of neutrophils EXCEPT

A: acid phosphatase.
B: elastase.
C: glycogen.
D: cathepsin.
E: collagenase.

Learning Response C: Correct. Glycogen is stored in the cytoplasm of neutrophils.

126. SUBJECT AREA: Blood and Myeloid Tissue
QUESTION: In females, the inactive X chromosome of neutrophils

A: cannot normally be distinguished in blood smears.
B: can only be seen by electron microscopy.
C: forms a drumstick-like appendage on one of the nuclear lobes.
D: forms one of the major lobes of the nucleus.
E: is one of the strands of nuclear material that exists between the nuclear lobes.

Learning Response C: Correct. The inactive X chromosome or Barr body forms an appendage of one of the lobes of the neutrophil nucleus.

127. SUBJECT AREA: Blood and Myeloid Tissue
QUESTION: Human erythrocytes

A: are removed from circulation by macrophages in the spleen and bone marrow.
B: retain their complement of mitochondria for their entire life-span in the peripheral blood circulation.
C: known as reticulocytes can increase in number in peripheral circulation as a result of hemorrhage.

    D: with diameters greater than 9 µm are known
       as microcytes.
    E: are characterized by choices A and C above.

Learning Response E: Correct. Mature red blood cells lose most of their organelles prior to entering the peripheral circulation. Those cells with diameters greater than 9 µm are called macrocytes; those with diameters less than 6 µm are known as microcytes.

---

128. SUBJECT AREA: Blood and Myeloid Tissue
       QUESTION: All of the following leukocytes are terminally
         differentiated EXCEPT

    A: basophils.
    B: eosinophils.
    C: neutrophils.
    D: monocytes.
    E: microphages.

Learning Response D: Correct. Monocytes can differentiate into macrophages in connective tissue and osteoclasts in bone. Neutrophils are also known as microphages because of their phagocytic activity and relatively smaller size than macrophages.

---

129. SUBJECT AREA: Blood and Myeloid Tissue
       QUESTION: Basophils

    A: neutralize bacterial toxins by the secretion
       of lysozyme.
    B: have granules which contain arylsulfatase.
    C: migrate from the peripheral blood stream to the
       connective tissues.
    D: are cytochemically and pharmacologically similar
       to mast cells.
    E: constitute approximately 5% of the
       circulating leukocytes.

Learning Response D: Correct. Basophils, which form less than 1% of the blood leukocytes, have granules which contain heparin and histamine and function similarly to mast cells in connective tissue. Basophils do not normally leave the blood stream. Lysozyme is a component of the specific granules of neutrophils.

---

130. SUBJECT AREA: Blood and Myeloid Tissue

QUESTION: B lymphocytes exhibit all of the following features EXCEPT that they

A: originate from stem cells in red bone marrow.

B: differentiate into plasma cells in connective tissue.

C: can be assisted by helper T cells to act against foreign antigens.

D: can be distinguished from T lymphocytes in hematoxylin and eosin (H&E) stained preparations.

E: function in the immunological marking of bacterial cells for destruction.

Learning Response D: Correct. In normal histological preparations, B lymphocytes are indistinguishable from T cells by H&E staining. Immunocytochemical techniques use antibodies to specific surface glycoproteins as a means of differentiating these two populations of cells.

---

131. SUBJECT AREA: Blood and Myeloid Tissue

QUESTION: Which of the following statements about T lymphocytes is NOT correct?

A: The specific type of cell surface receptor on T lymphocytes is one of the classes of immunoglobulin molecules.

B: Cytotoxic T cells secrete substances which attack tumor cells or virus infected cells.

C: T lymphocytes originate in red bone marrow but mature in the thymus.

D: T lymphocytes can recognize foreign antigens and can elaborate lymphokines (interleukins) which affect the activity of other cells.

E: T lymphocytes can act as suppressors of the
immune response.

Learning Response A: Correct. T lymphocytes have T cell receptors as their
specific type of surface glycoprotein which distinguishes them from B
lymphocytes which have immunoglobulin surface proteins.

---

132. SUBJECT AREA: Blood and Myeloid Tissue
QUESTION: Neutrophils or polymorphonuclear leukocytes

A: have a nucleus that consists of 2-5 lobes.
B: are the largest of the leukocytes.
C: are the most numerous of the circulating
leukocytes.
D: are characterized by choices A and C only.
E: have all of the above features.

Learning Response D: Correct. Neutrophils constitute approximately 60-70%
of the leukocytes in the peripheral circulation and have a multilobed nucleus.
Their average diameter is less than that of monocytes which are the largest of
the leukocytes in the peripheral blood stream.

---

133. SUBJECT AREA: Blood and Myeloid Tissue
QUESTION: Which of the following statements about platelets is
NOT correct?

A: In red bone marrow, platelets develop from part
of the cytoplasm of a megakaryocyte.
B: The external cell coat of glycosaminoglycans aids
in platelet adhesion.
C: Platelets are 2-4 μm in diameter and have a life-
span of approximately 60 days.
D: Platelets contain lysosomal enzymes and platelet-
derived growth factor in separate populations
of granules.
E: The activation of platelets involves the extension of
filopodia containing actin microfilaments.

Learning Response C: Correct. The normal life-span of platelets in the peripheral blood stream is about 10 days.

134. SUBJECT AREA: Blood and Myeloid Tissue

QUESTION: An erythrocyte normally enters all of the following developmental stages in bone marrow EXCEPT

   A: polychromatophilic erythroblast.
   B: proerythroblast.
   C: reticulocyte.
   D: myelocyte.
   E: basophilic erythroblast.

Learning Response D: Correct. Myelocytes are a stage of leukocyte differentiation.

135. SUBJECT AREA: Blood and Myeloid Tissue

QUESTION: In the bone marrow, the first recognizable cell in the differentiation of granulocytes is the

   A: promyelocyte stage.
   B: myelocyte stage.
   C: metamyelocyte stage.
   D: band form.
   E: myeloblast stage.

Learning Response E: Correct. The first recognizable cell in the differentiation of granulocytic leukocytes appears in the myeloblast stage.

136. SUBJECT AREA: Blood and Myeloid Tissue

QUESTION: Which of the following statements about hematopoiesis is NOT correct?

   A: In the adult, hematopoiesis normally occurs in the spleen and liver, as well as in the bone marrow.
   B: The primordial or prehepatic phase can begin as early as the third week of embryonic life.

C: It is initiated in the embryo by elongated clusters of mesenchymal cells in the yolk sac.

D: It becomes centered in the liver by the third month of embryonic life.

E: It occurs almost exclusively in the bone marrow after the sixth month of embryonic life.

Learning Response A: Correct. The liver and spleen function as blood forming organs only during embryonic life.

137. SUBJECT AREA: Blood and Myeloid Tissue
QUESTION: Which of the following cell types are stem cells?

A: skeletal muscle cells
B: metamyelocytes
C: colony forming cells (CFCs)
D: mast cells
E: neutrophils

Learning Response C: Correct. Key features of stem cells include their potentiality and their self-renewing capacity. Of the choices listed, only colony forming cells in bone marrow exhibit these characteristics.

138. SUBJECT AREA: Blood and Myeloid Tissue
QUESTION: Megakaryocytes

A: are located in red bone marrow.
B: give rise to platelets by fragmentation of their cytoplasm.
C: are relatively small cells with lobulated nuclei.
D: are characterized by choices A and B above.
E: are characterized by choices A, B and C above.

Learning Response D: Correct. Megakaryocytes are large cells (between 30-150 μm in diameter), are located in bone marrow and produce platelets by the shedding of cytoplasm.

139. SUBJECT AREA: Blood and Myeloid Tissue
QUESTION: Lymphocytes which circulate in the peripheral
blood stream

A: originate from progenitor cells in the bone marrow
and complete their maturation elsewhere.
B: consist only of T lymphocytes; B lymphocytes are
restricted to the lymphoid tissues and organs.
C: originate from lymphoblasts which are the last cells
in the developmental series to exhibit mitosis.
D: consist only of B lymphocytes; T lymphocytes are
restricted to the lymphoid organs.
E: migrate into the same compartments within
lymphoid tissues.

Learning Response A: Correct. Progenitor cells in the bone marrow produce
cells which gain immunological competence in the primary or central
lymphoid organs. Both T and B cells are found in the peripheral circulation
and can migrate to lymphoid organs where they populate distinct
compartments.

140. SUBJECT AREA: Blood and Myeloid Tissue
QUESTION: Monocytes

A: are derived from monoblasts and promonocytes
in the bone marrow.
B: circulate in peripheral blood for about 8 hours and
then migrate to connective tissue.
C: mature into phagocytic macrophages which can
function for several months.
D: contain small cytoplasmic granules which
are primary lysosomes.
E: exhibit all of the above features.

Learning Response E: Correct. Monocytes begin their development in the
bone marrow and migrate to connective tissues where they terminally
differentiate into macrophages.

141. SUBJECT AREA: Blood and Myeloid Tissue

QUESTION: Bone marrow has all of the following features EXCEPT that

A: it is located in the medullary canals of long bones.

B: it is the major site of blood cell formation.

C: in newborns it consists of a mixture of red and yellow marrow.

D: under certain conditions can be converted from yellow marrow to red.

E: it is located in the cavities of spongy or cancellous bone.

Learning Response C: Correct. In newborn infants all of the bone marrow is red and active in hematopoiesis.

142. SUBJECT AREA: Blood and Myeloid Tissue

QUESTION: Which of the following statements is NOT characteristic of red bone marrow?

A: The connective tissue stroma of red marrow consists of reticular fibers in which the hematopoietic cells are embedded.

B: A special type of matrix protein called laminin binds the developing blood cells to the matrix fibers.

C: Mature blood cells migrate through the walls of sinusoidal capillaries into the peripheral circulation.

D: Releasing factors that include hormones and bacterial toxins control the movement of blood cells from the red marrow.

E: In addition to hematopoiesis, red marrow also functions in the destruction of erythrocytes.

Learning Response B: Correct. The cell binding matrix protein called hemonectin interacts with blood cells to attach them to the matrix.

143. SUBJECT AREA: Blood and Myeloid Tissue

QUESTION: All of the following are true about neutrophilic precursors EXCEPT that they

A: produce the most common type of leukocyte in peripheral circulation.

B: are normally restricted to red bone marrow.

C: produce cells which can migrate from the blood to connective tissue.

D: secrete immunoglobulin A molecules.

E: produce cells which function in the destruction of bacterial cells.

Learning Response D: Correct. Neither neutrophils nor their precursors synthesize and secrete immunoglobulins.

144. SUBJECT AREA: Blood and Myeloid Tissue

QUESTION: All of the following occur in the development of erythrocytes EXCEPT

A: an increase in cytoplasmic basophilia.

B: a decrease in cell size.

C: a decrease in the numbers of mitochondria.

D: a decrease in the size of the nucleolus.

E: a decrease in nuclear diameter.

Learning Response A: Correct. In the stages of erythrocyte development from basophilic erythroblast to mature red blood cell, the numbers of polyribosomes decrease as less synthesis of proteins occurs. The lack of polyribosomes corresponds to a decrease in cytoplasmic basophilia.

145. SUBJECT AREA: Blood and Myeloid Tissue

QUESTION: The orthochromatophilic erythroblast

A: has a euchromatic nucleus.

B: exhibits an acidophilic cytoplasm similar to that of mature cells.

C: is generally much larger in size than the
   mature cell.
D: usually has two nucleoli.
E: is normally found in the peripheral circulation.

Learning Response B: Correct. The orthochromatophilic erythroblast is the stage of development just prior to the reticulocyte which is an anucleate cell. The orthochromatophilic erythroblast has lost much of its polyribosomes, and as a result its cytoplasm is acidophilic and is packed with hemoglobin. The cell is approximately the same size as the mature red blood cell.

---

146. SUBJECT AREA: Blood and Myeloid Tissue
       QUESTION: The first recognizable cell in the erythroid
                developmental series is the

A: reticulocyte.
B: polychromatophilic erythroblast.
C: basophilic erythroblast.
D: proerythroblast.
E: erythrocyte colony forming progenitor cell.

Learning Response D: Correct. Choices A to D are recognizable cells in the bone marrow. The earliest cell in this series is the proerythroblast which is a large cell with a euchromatic nucleus and nucleoli. Its cytoplasm is basophilic. The erythrocyte colony forming cell is not distinguishable from those of the leukocyte and megakaryocyte series.

---

147. SUBJECT AREA: Blood and Myeloid Tissue
       QUESTION: In the development of granulocytes, the first signs
                of differentiation occur at the _____ stage.

A: metamyelocyte
B: promyelocyte
C: myelocyte
D: band cell
E: mature cell

Learning Response C: Correct. Promyelocytes divide to form neutrophilic, eosinophilic and basophilic myelocytes. Thus, the myelocyte stage is the first stage of recognizable differentiation.

---

148. SUBJECT AREA: Blood and Myeloid Tissue
QUESTION: In the development of neutrophils, the cells pass through several compartments which include

    A: medullary storage compartment, capable of releasing large numbers of mature cells.
    B: circulating compartment in which the cells are in the blood plasma.
    C: medullary formation compartment in which mitosis and maturation occur.
    D: marginating compartment in which the cells, although present in blood, are held temporarily in capillaries.
    E: all of the above compartments.

Learning Response E: Correct. Immature and mature cells in the neutrophilic cell series can appear in all of the above compartments prior to their migration from blood into connective tissue.

---

149. SUBJECT AREA: Cartilage
QUESTION: Cartilage

    A: has more glycosaminoglycan and more collagen than does bone.
    B: capping of the articular surfaces of long bones is nourished by diffusion from its perichondrium.
    C: has a smaller proportion of hyaluronic acid than bone.
    D: only grows by interstitial cell division.
    E: contains different types of connective tissue fibers depending on the support being provided.

Learning Response E: Correct. There are three types of cartilage: hyaline cartilage, elastic cartilage and fibrocartilage. They are characterized by the variation in the composition of their matrix components. Articular cartilage lacks a perichondrium. Cartilage grows by division of cells in the perichondrium (appositional growth) and by division of cells in the matrix (interstitial growth). Much of this growth occurs during early development. Cartilage in the mature adult is postmitotic.

150. SUBJECT AREA: Cartilage
QUESTION: All of the following macromolecules are found in cartilage EXCEPT

A: glycosaminoglycans.
B: collagen.
C: hyaluronic acid.
D: hydroxyapatite crystals.
E: proteoglycans.

Learning Response D: Correct. Hydroxyapatite crystals are found in bone matrix.

151. SUBJECT AREA: Cartilage
QUESTION: Type I collagen fibers are found in

A: fibrocartilage.
B: hyaline cartilage.
C: elastic cartilage.
D: choices A and B above.
E: hyaline cartilage and bone.

Learning Response A: Correct. Fibrocartilage contains a dense network of coarse type I collagen fibers. It is found in regions of the body subjected to great stress in weight bearing areas.

152. SUBJECT AREA: Cartilage
QUESTION: The perichondrium

A: is avascular.
B: is found covering every cartilage surface.
C: is a loose connective tissue lining cartilage.

D: is essential for the growth and maintenance
   of cartilage.
E: has a cellular layer in which the cells eventually
   convert to osteocytes.

Learning Response D: Correct. The perichondrium consists of dense
connective tissue that lines cartilage. It contains blood vessels which supply
nourishment for the avascular cartilage tissue. Cartilage at the surface of
bones (articular cartilage) and fibrocartilage are devoid of a perichondrium.

153. SUBJECT AREA: Cartilage
QUESTION: Hyaline cartilage

A: contains lymphatic vessels and nerve fibers.
B: is vascularized.
C: always converts to bone in the adult.
D: contains chondrocytes that exhibit a high metabolic
   activity.
E: serves as a temporary skeleton in the embryo.

Learning Response E: Correct. Hyaline cartilage is avascular and is
nourished from the capillaries in the perichondrium or synovial fluid. It does
not have lymphatic vessels or nerves. Chondrocytes exhibit a low metabolic
activity due to the tissue's avascularity, and hence, hyaline cartilage features a
slow rate of healing after injury.

154. SUBJECT AREA: Cartilage
QUESTION: Cartilage proteoglycans

A: chondroitin sulfate side chains are electrostatically
   bound to the collagen fibrils.
B: are made up of 85% of their dry weight by
   chondroitin sulfates.
C: contain keratan sulfate.
D: are noncovalently associated with molecules
   of hyaluronic acid.
E: exhibit all of the above characteristics.

Learning Response E: Correct. Cartilage proteoglycans consist of chondroitin-4-sulfate, chondroitin-6-sulfate and keratan sulfate glycosaminoglycans, all of which are covalently linked to a protein core.

155. SUBJECT AREA: Cartilage
QUESTION: Chondrocytes

A: that are still immature are round with little or no surface indentations or protrusions.
B: that have matured, contain only a few organelles which are necessary to maintain their own survival.
C: synthesize type IV collagen.
D: have finger-like projections connecting one cell to another by gap junctions.
E: are immediately surrounded by an area called the territorial matrix.

Learning Response E: Correct. Mature chondrocytes have a large amount of rough endoplasmic reticulum and a well developed Golgi complex in order to synthesize type II collagen, proteoglycans and chondronectin. The area immediately surrounding the chondrocytes, the territorial matrix, is rich in glycosaminoglycans and low in collagen.

156. SUBJECT AREA: Cartilage
QUESTION: A cartilage cell's

A: function is retarded by growth hormone, thyroxine and testosterone.
B: function is accelerated by cortisone, hydrocortisone and estradiol.
C: growth depends upon blood calcium levels.
D: growth has a direct dependency on the hypophyseal growth hormone, somatotropin.
E: mutation can give rise to malignant tumors known as chondrosarcoma.

Learning Response E: Correct. Growth hormone, thyroxine and testosterone accelerate chondrocyte function where cortisone, hydrocortisone and estradiol retard function. Somatotropin does not act directly on cartilage cells. It does, however, promote the synthesis of somatomedin C in the liver which acts directly on chondrocytes to promote their growth.

---

157. SUBJECT AREA: Cartilage
QUESTION: Appositional growth

> *A:* results from the mitotic division of chondrocytes.
> *B:* results from the differentiation of perichondrial cells.
> *C:* occurs at a slower rate than that of interstitial growth.
> *D:* increases tissue mass by expanding the cartilage matrix from within.
> *E:* occurs in the epiphyseal plates of long bones.

Learning Response B: Correct. Chondroblasts of the perichondrium proliferate and become chondrocytes after they are surrounded with cartilaginous matrix. Appositional growth is a more rapid growth than interstitial growth. In both cases, chondrocytes synthesize collagen fibrils and ground substance. Appositional growth can occur during regeneration of damaged cartilage.

---

158. SUBJECT AREA: Cartilage
QUESTION: What type of cartilage is depicted in the figure below?

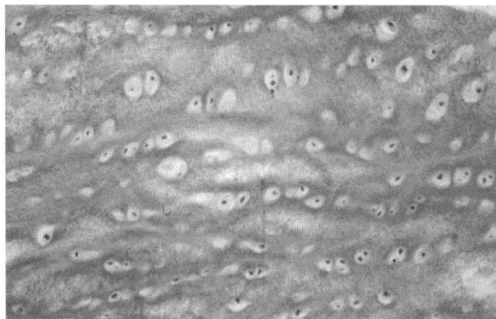

> *A:* hyaline cartilage
> *B:* proliferative zone of the epiphyseal plate

C: fibrocartilage
D: elastic cartilage
E: articular cartilage

Learning Response C: Correct. Fibrocartilage has rows of chondrocytes separated by an abundant amount of type I collagen fibers and lacks a perichondrium. This type of cartilage is found mainly in intervertebral disks and in the pubic symphysis.

---

159. SUBJECT AREA: Cartilage
QUESTION: Elastic cartilage is identical to hyaline cartilage EXCEPT that it

A: contains type I collagen.
B: contains an abundant amount of fine elastic fibers.
C: does not have a perichondrium.
D: has a lower percentage of proteoglycans in its matrix.
E: does not contain the glycoprotein chondronectin.

Learning Response B: Correct. Elastic cartilage contains a predominant amount of fine elastic fibers, type II collagen and all the same components in its matrix as does hyaline cartilage. Elastic cartilage is found in the auricle of the ear, in the wall of the external auditory canals, in the eustachian tubes, the epiglottis and the cuneiform cartilage of the larynx.

---

160. SUBJECT AREA: Cartilage
QUESTION: Where would one find the type of cartilage depicted in the figure below?

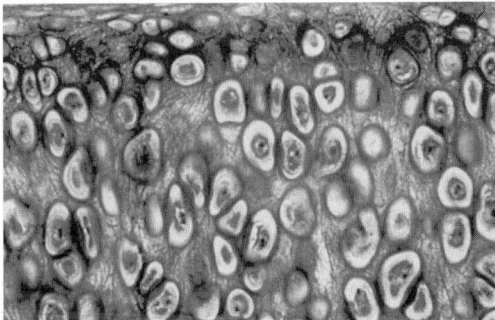

A: trachea
B: epiphyseal plate of bone
C: intervertebral disk
D: symphysis pubis
E: epiglottis

Learning Response E: Correct. The figure is a photomicrograph of elastic cartilage. This tissue can be found in the epiglottis and the auricle of the ear. The epiphyseal plate consists of hyaline cartilage. Fibrocartilage can be found in intervertebral disks and the symphysis pubis.

161. SUBJECT AREA: Cartilage
QUESTION: The major role of hyaline cartilage in the adult human is

A: in the development of long bones.
B: flexible support of the external ear.
C: in blood production.
D: to provide a shock absorber in joints.
E: to provide resistance to stretching of the symphysis pubis.

Learning Response D: Correct. Hyaline cartilage is found at the articular surface of long bones and it absorbs much of the shock transmitted to the bones by their movements.

162. SUBJECT AREA: Cartilage
QUESTION: Fibrocartilage can be defined as a combination of

A: hyaline cartilage and bone.
B: hyaline cartilage and dense connective tissue.
C: elastic cartilage and bone.
D: elastic cartilage and dense connective tissue.
E: hyaline cartilage and loose connective tissue.

Learning Response B: Correct. Fibrocartilage has characteristics which are intermediate between those of hyaline cartilage and dense connective tissue. The tissue contains chondrocytes similar to those in hyaline cartilage and type I collagen fibers similar to those in dense connective tissue.

163. SUBJECT AREA: Cartilage
  QUESTION: Feature(s) consistent with both fibrocartilage and
  articular cartilage include(s)

  A: absence of a perichondrium.
  B: presence of cells in lacunae.
  C: presence of collagen fibers in the matrix.
  D: choices A, B and C above.
  E: choices B and C above.

Learning Response D: Correct. Articular cartilage and fibrocartilage share a number of features. Both lack a perichondrium. Their cells reside in lacunae and collagen fibrils are found in the matrix. In articular cartilage these are type II collagen; in fibrocartilage, type I collagen.

164. SUBJECT AREA: Bone
  QUESTION: The following are all found in bone EXCEPT

  A: hydroxyapatite crystals.
  B: Howship's lacunae.
  C: type II collagen.
  D: Volkmann's canals.
  E: Sharpey's fibers.

Learning Response C: Correct. Type II collagen is the principal collagen found in hyaline cartilage. Both type I collagen and hydroxyapatite crystals are found in bone matrix. Howship's lacunae are depressions in the bone matrix which has been enzymatically etched out by the osteoclasts. Sharpey's fibers are bundles of collagen that bind the periosteum to bone. Haversian canals are connected by the Volkmann's canals.

165. SUBJECT AREA: Bone
  QUESTION: A function of osteoclasts is

  A: resorption and remodeling of bone.
  B: synthesizing bone matrix.
  C: forming canaliculi in bone.

D: to differentiate into osteocytes after bone matrix
    has calcified.
E: to perform all of the above functions.

Learning Response A: Correct. Osteoclasts are multinucleated giant cells
that are involved in the resorption and remodeling of bone tissue. They are
derived from blood monocytes.

---

166. SUBJECT AREA: Bone
    QUESTION: Which one of the following methods is best used when
        preparing bone for light microscopic viewing?

    A: microtome sectioning
    B: slicing bone with a tissue chopper
    C: grinding slices of bone with abrasives
    D: sectioning bone with a hand saw
    E: freeze fracture

Learning Response C: Correct. Due to the hardness of bone, it is very
difficult to section on a microtome or tissue chopper. Slices are ground
using abrasives until they are thin enough to be translucent. Another
method used for bone observation is decalcification, embedding in paraffin or
plastic, sectioning and staining with an appropriate dye such as hematoxylin
and eosin.

---

167. SUBJECT AREA: Bone
    QUESTION: Bone canaliculi

    A: are formed by enzymatic activity of
        osteoclasts.
    B: are cytoplasmic extensions of osteoid.
    C: are channel-like structures which house
        cytoplasmic extensions of osteocytes.
    D: can be seen using a silver stain.
    E: connect Haversian canals to one another.

Learning Response C: Correct. Canaliculi are thin spaces that are formed around osteoblast cytoplasmic processes as the bone matrix is being laid down.

---

168. SUBJECT AREA: Bone
        QUESTION: Within the lacunae of bone, there are

> *A:* osteoprogenitor cells.
> *B:* osteoblasts which are capable of undergoing mitosis.
> *C:* blood vessels and nerves.
> *D:* fibroblast cells.
> *E:* osteocytes.

Learning Response E: Correct. Only one osteocyte, incapable of undergoing mitosis, is found in each lacuna. The osteocyte is active in maintaining the bone matrix.

---

169. SUBJECT AREA: Bone
        QUESTION: In bone,

> *A:* type I collagen fibers are arranged in the same manner in compact and woven (immature) bone.
> *B:* osteoclasts are found only on the periosteal surfaces.
> *C:* Haversian systems are interconnected by Haversian canals.
> *D:* osteoclasts have surface modifications similar to cilia that aid in the movement of calcium toward blood vessels.
> *E:* both endochondral and intramembranous ossification produce woven bone.

Learning Response E: Correct. Intramembranous ossification takes place within clusters of mesenchymal cells. Endochondral ossification occurs within a skeletal model formed by hyaline cartilage. Both types of ossification produce immature or woven bone.

170. SUBJECT AREA: Bone

QUESTION: In bone,

A: circumferential lamellae can become interstitial
lamellae as a result of remodeling.

B: only osteoblasts and osteocytes are required for
normal bone resorption.

C: osteocytes are connected by tight junctions.

D: remodeling can only occur at the endosteal
surfaces of bone.

E: Volkmann's canals are formed by the action of
lysosomal enzymes after osteoid has calcified.

Learning Response A: Correct. During the growth of bone, there is a
continuous destruction and rebuilding of Haversian systems. Osteoclasts are
necessary for bone resorption.

171. SUBJECT AREA: Bone

QUESTION: All of the following characteristics are true about bone
EXCEPT that

A: cancellous bone is the target for resorption if blood
calcium levels fall too low.

B: hydrogen ion secretion is an essential component of
osteoclastic activity.

C: Haversian systems are lined by osteoprogenitor
cells and osteoclasts.

D: circumferential lamellae surround the entire bone.

E: the periosteum is the site of appositional
bone growth.

Learning Response C: Correct. Haversian systems are lined by endosteum.
Bone lining cells in the endosteum can function as osteoprogenitor cells.

172. SUBJECT AREA: Bone

QUESTION: Interstitial lamellae are

A: the outer lamellae of osteons.
B: remnants of old osteons.
C: lamellae surrounding Volkmann's canals.
D: lamellae at the periphery of bone.
E: newly formed lamellae.

Learning Response B: Correct. Interstitial lamellae represent lamellae left by Haversian systems destroyed during growth and remodeling of bone.

---

173. SUBJECT AREA: Bone
QUESTION: Sources of osteoblasts are

A: osteocytes.
B: chondrocytes.
C: osteoclasts.
D: monocytes that migrated from the blood.
E: periosteal osteoprogenitor cells.

Learning Response E: Correct. Progenitor cells in the periosteum and bone lining cells in the endosteum are sources of osteoblasts. Osteoclasts are derived from monocytes which migrated into bone from the blood.

---

174. SUBJECT AREA: Bone
QUESTION: In endochondral ossification,

A: chondrocytes differentiate into osteoblasts.
B: chondrocytes respond to the absence of nutrients by calcifying the matrix.
C: osteogenesis occurs in the absence of a vascular supply.
D: osteoclasts do not function until cancellous bone is changed to compact bone.
E: the zone of proliferation is characterized by an enlargement of the chondrocytes.

Learning Response B: Correct. The presence of a collar of bone surrounding the cartilage prevents the diffusion of nutrients into the cartilage. As a result, the chondrocytes degenerate and their matrix becomes calcified.

---

175. SUBJECT AREA: Bone

QUESTION: Which of the following statements about intramembranous ossification is NOT correct?

A: Osteoblasts are surrounded by osteoid matrix prior to calcification.

B: Bone develops in clusters of mesenchymal cells.

C: Cells in the outermost layer of the perichondrium are the osteoprogenitor cells.

D: Osteoclasts remodel the newly formed bone.

E: Osteogenesis results primarily in the formation of the flat bones of the skull.

Learning Response C: Correct. Intramembranous ossification occurs in the absence of a cartilaginous model, and, thus, there is no perichondrium.

---

176. SUBJECT AREA: Bone

QUESTION: In the figure below of the epiphyseal plate, what process is occurring in the hypertrophic cartilage zone?

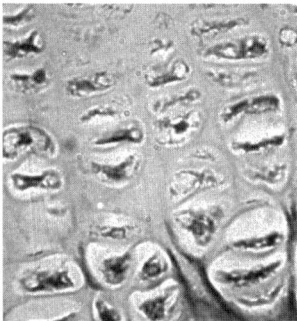

A: Chondrocytes are preparing to divide.

B: Chondrocytes are beginning to accumulate glycogen.

C: Cell death is occurring due to calcification of the matrix.

D: Bone tissue is beginning to form.

E: Osteocytes are actively dividing and forming rows.

Learning Response B: Correct. In the hypertrophic cartilage zone, the cells are beginning to increase in size due to glycogen accumulation. There is little matrix between the chrondrocytes.

---

177. SUBJECT AREA: Bone

QUESTION: When comparing primary bone verses secondary bone,

A: primary bone has an irregular array of collagen fibers whereas secondary bone has collagen fibers arranged in lamellae.

B: primary bone has a lower proportion of osteocytes per μm^3 than secondary bone.

C: primary bone has a higher mineral content than secondary bone.

D: primary bone can be found only in embryos and not in adults; secondary bone can be found only in adults.

E: all of the statements are correct.

Learning Response A: Correct. Primary bone has a higher proportion of osteocytes per μm^3 than secondary bone, and has less mineral content. Primary bone is formed in embryos as well as adults.

---

178. SUBJECT AREA: Bone

QUESTION: All of the following statements are true about Haversian systems or osteons EXCEPT that

A: the central canal is surrounded by 4-20 concentric lamellae.

B: in each lamella, collagen fibers run parallel to each other.

C: the central canal contains blood vessels and nerves.

D: endosteum lines the inner surface.

E: the cementing substance is found between each lamella in the Haversian system.

Learning Response E: Correct. Cementing substance is an amorphous material that consists of mineralized matrix with few collagen fibers. It is found surrounding each Haversian system, not between each lamella.

---

179. SUBJECT AREA: Bone

QUESTION: When bone is fractured,

A: osteoprogenitor cells proliferate intensely around the break.

B: primary bone is formed by endochondral ossification of small cartilage fragments.

C: bone is formed by intramembranous ossification.

D: primary bone of the callus is gradually resorbed and replaced by secondary bone.

E: all of the above events occur.

Learning Response E: Correct. Destruction of bone matrix and cell death occur when a bone is fractured. During repair, macrophages remove dead and damaged cells. Osteoprogenitor cells of the periosteum and the endosteum proliferate to form a cellular tissue surrounding and penetrating the fractured bone. Primary bone is then formed by endochondral ossification. Bone is also formed by intramembranous ossification. This results in a bone callus. The bone callus is gradually resorbed and replaced by secondary bone restoring it to its original bone structure.

---

180. SUBJECT AREA: Bone

QUESTION: Osteoporosis

A: is a nutritional deficiency.

B: is caused by a decrease in the amount of calcium per unit of bone matrix.

C: is a decrease in bone mass caused by decreased bone formation and/or increased resorption.

D: is usually found in female children and postmenopausal women.

E: can be characterized by all of the above statements.

Learning Response C: Correct. Osteoporosis is not a nutritional deficiency as is osteomalacia. Osteoporosis occurs in immobilized patients and postmenopausal women.

---

181. SUBJECT AREA: Bone
QUESTION: Diarthroses are joints that

> *A:* lack connective tissue capsules.
> *B:* are joined by hyaline cartilage.
> *C:* are joined by an interosseous ligament of dense connective tissue.
> *D:* have great mobility.
> *E:* are continually remodeled due to the deterioration of the hyaline cartilage.

Learning Response D: Correct. Synostoses are joints in which no movement takes place. Synchondroses are articulations which bones are connected by hyaline cartilage, and syndesmoses are joints that allow a certain amount of movement and are joined by an interosseous ligament of dense connective tissue. Diarthroses are enclosed by a dense connective tissue capsule.

---

182. SUBJECT AREA: Bone
QUESTION: In the figure below, identify the cell labelled by the arrow.

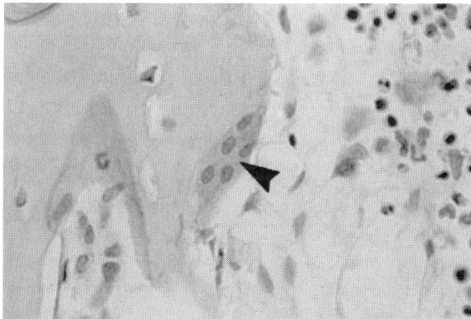

> *A:* macrophage
> *B:* fibroblast

C: osteoclast
D: cell of the diffuse neuroendocrine system
E: osteoblast

Learning Response C: Correct. Large multinucleated cells adjacent to bone are osteoclasts which function in bone remodeling. None of the other cells in the list of choices is multinucleated.

---

183. SUBJECT AREA: Bone
QUESTION: Articular cartilage

A: is hyaline cartilage without a perichondrium.
B: is found lining joints of long bones.
C: absorbs the mechanical pressures of joints.
D: has collagen fibers that run first perpendicular and then parallel to the cartilage surface.
E: has all of the above characteristics.

Learning Response E: Correct. Articular cartilage is a smooth, friction-free layer of hyaline cartilage lining joints of long bones. It persists throughout adult life and does not contribute to bone formation.

---

184. SUBJECT AREA: Bone
QUESTION: The synovial membrane

A: has no basal lamina between the lining cells and the underlying connective tissue.
B: is avascular.
C: contains large amounts of adipose cells.
D: has an internal layer of columnar cells.
E: has cells which are connected by tight junctions.

Learning Response A: Correct. The synovial membrane is highly vascularized with some areas of adipose tissue. Its internal layer is lined with squamous or cuboidal cells.

185. SUBJECT AREA: Muscle Tissue

QUESTION: The thin filament proteins involved in the calcium regulation of contraction in striated muscle are

A: actin and myosin.
B: troponin and tropomyosin.
C: myosin and tropomyosin.
D: calsequestrin and troponin.
E: calsequestrin and actin.

Learning Response B: Correct. Calcium binds to the TnC subunit of troponin which is a complex of three subunits bound to the thin filament by tropomyosin.

186. SUBJECT AREA: Muscle Tissue

QUESTION: In the sarcomere, the ATPase required for contraction is localized in the

A: sarcoplasmic reticulum.
B: thin filaments.
C: thick and thin filaments.
D: myosin heads or crossbridges.
E: actin-tropomyosin-troponin complex.

Learning Response D: Correct. Myosin has both enzymatic activity and the ability to bind to actin to produce a shortening of the sarcomere.

187. SUBJECT AREA: Muscle Tissue

QUESTION: Smooth muscle cells

A: lack intermediate filaments.
B: have an elaborate network of sarcoplasmic reticulum.
C: have large diameter transverse tubules.
D: require calcium ions as activators of myosin-actin interactions.
E: form a syncytium similar to skeletal muscle.

Learning Response D: Correct. Smooth muscle cells lack troponin but require calcium for their contractile activity. Calcium activates an enzyme which phosphorylates the light chain of myosin allowing myosin to bind to actin and hydrolyze ATP. All three types of muscle have intermediate filaments. Smooth muscle lacks transverse tubules and consists of single cells with little extracellular matrix.

---

188. SUBJECT AREA: Muscle Tissue

QUESTION: Which structural features would allow you to distinguish skeletal from cardiac and smooth muscle?

A: presence of organized thick and thin filaments
B: location of nuclei in the fiber
C: presence of a sarcoplasmic reticulum
D: localization of troponin in thin filaments
E: presence of intermediate filaments

Learning Response B: Correct. Cardiac and smooth muscle cells have centrally located nuclei in contrast to skeletal muscle cells which have their nuclei in a peripheral location.

---

189. SUBJECT AREA: Muscle Tissue

QUESTION: Which of the following statements about the motor end-plate or myoneural junction is NOT correct?

A: Acetylcholine receptors are present in the specialized basal lamina.
B: The sarcolemma forms junctional folds.
C: The muscle fiber basal lamina surrounds the Schwann cell.
D: Acetylcholine is released by exocytosis.
E: The axon terminal is unmyelinated.

Learning Response A: Correct. Acetylcholine receptors are located in the sarcolemma of the junctional folds of the skeletal muscle cell.

190. SUBJECT AREA: Muscle Tissue
QUESTION: An antibody that binds to the globular head (S1) of striated muscle myosin

    A: would localize throughout the A band.
    B: would localize at the M line.
    C: would localize in the I band.
    D: may alter the interaction of myosin with actin.
    E: would most likely affect the formation of thick filaments.

Learning Response D: Correct. The heads of myosin molecules extend out from the thick myofilaments to interact with actin in the thin filaments. Antibody binding in this region would affect this interaction. The heads of myosin are not found throughout the A band and are absent from the M line area. The tails of myosin molecules would be found throughout the entire thick filament. Antibody binding would be absent from the I bands since this region contains only actin filaments.

191. SUBJECT AREA: Muscle Tissue
QUESTION: In comparing myosin I with myosin II,

    A: both proteins function as membrane translocators.
    B: both proteins can bind only one molecule of ATP.
    C: both proteins are located in nonmuscle cells.
    D: myosin light chain kinase phosphorylates both proteins.
    E: myosin I is found in the thick filaments of smooth muscle cells, and myosin II is the major protein in the thick filaments of striated muscle cells.

Learning Response C: Correct. Both proteins are present in nonmuscle cells. Myosin I functions as a membrane translocator by binding to actin and to membrane phospholipids. Myosin I binds one molecule of ATP, the hydrolysis of which provides the energy for its activity. Myosin II forms short bipolar filaments in nonmuscle cells and by binding to actin and hydrolyzing

ATP accounts for movements in nonmuscle cells. Myosin II, because of its two globular heads, can bind two ATP molecules. Myosin light chain kinase phosphorylates myosin II in nonmuscle cells and in smooth muscle cells allowing the myosin to form filaments.

---

192. SUBJECT AREA: Muscle Tissue

QUESTION: All of the following statements about smooth muscle are true EXCEPT that they

A: are elongated, spindle-shaped cells.
B: lack tropomyosin and troponin.
C: can synthesize the proteins of connective tissue.
D: are controlled by the autonomic nervous system.
E: contain intermediate filaments.

Learning Response B: Correct. Smooth muscle cells possess tropomyosin which functions as an actin binding protein, but lack troponin which functions in calcium regulation in striated muscle. In smooth muscle, calcium regulation occurs through the calcium dependent phosphorylation of myosin by the enzyme myosin light chain kinase. Smooth muscle cells in the walls of large elastic arteries and elsewhere have the ability to synthesize and secrete connective tissue proteins.

---

193. SUBJECT AREA: Muscle Tissue

QUESTION: All of the following are features of cardiac muscle EXCEPT

A: the presence of smooth endoplasmic reticulum.
B: the ability to regenerate following injury or trauma.
C: the presence of desmin containing intermediate filaments.
D: the presence of myofibrils.
E: the presence of innervation via the autonomic nervous system.

Learning Response B: Correct. When cardiac muscle cells are injured, the cells do not regenerate and die. They are replaced by scar tissue. Unlike skeletal muscle which has a population of undifferentiated cells (satellite cells) which have the ability to replace cells lost by trauma or injury, cardiac muscle lacks such primitive cells and, thus, cannot regenerate.

---

194. SUBJECT AREA: Muscle Tissue
QUESTION: In skeletal muscle, the triad

> *A:* is the site of excitation-contraction coupling.
> *B:* consists of a complex of myosin-actin-tropomyosin.
> *C:* consists of a transverse tubule flanked by two mitochondria.
> *D:* is a complex consisting of actin-tropomyosin-troponin.
> *E:* is usually located at the Z line in mammalian skeletal muscle.

Learning Response A: Correct. Muscle cells are stimulated to contract by action potentials generated in nerve fibers near the muscle cells. The resultant wave of depolarization is carried deep into the contractile apparatus by the transverse tubules which are flanked by two expanded regions of the sarcoplasmic reticulum known as terminal cisterns. The excitation of the muscle cell is coupled to its contractile activity at the triads which are usually located at the junction of A bands with I bands in mammalian muscle.

---

195. SUBJECT AREA: Muscle Tissue
QUESTION: Connective tissue which encases fascicles or bundles of skeletal muscle fibers is known as

> *A:* epimysium.
> *B:* perimysium.
> *C:* endomysium.
> *D:* basal lamina.
> *E:* basement membrane.

Learning Response B: Correct. Perimysial connective tissue which carries blood vessels and nerve fibers encloses bundles of skeletal muscle cells. Individual cells are surrounded by endomysium, a component of which is the basal lamina of the muscle cell. The entire muscle is encased by epimysium which contains the largest nerve fibers and blood vessels.

196. SUBJECT AREA: Muscle Tissue
QUESTION: All of the following statements about skeletal muscle
are true EXCEPT that

A: calcium ions are released through the junctional
feet of the sarcoplasmic reticulum.
B: the thick myofilaments remain constant in length as
the sarcomere shortens.
C: troponin binds calcium prior to myosin and actin
interactions in muscle contraction.
D: myosin crossbridges are permanently attached to
actin filaments in the absence of ATP.
E: calsequestrin is located in the longitudinal
component of the sarcoplasmic reticulum.

Learning Response E: Correct. Calsequestrin, the sarcoplasmic protein which
binds calcium in the absence of excitation and contraction, is located in the
dilated terminal cisterns of the sarcoplasmic reticulum. This assures the
proximity of calcium to the transverse tubules which carry the excitation
wave deep into the muscle cell.

197. SUBJECT AREA: Muscle Tissue
QUESTION: Smooth muscle cells

A: can be derived from all three germ layers:
endoderm, mesoderm or ectoderm.
B: are coupled by gap or communicating junctions
allowing the cells to contract as a sheet of tissue.
C: are the largest of the three types of muscle cells.
D: have an elaborate network of smooth endoplasmic
reticulum.
E: normally will not regenerate when injured.

Learning Response B: Correct. Unlike skeletal muscle which consists of a
morphological syncytium, smooth muscle is made up of individual cells
which function as a syncytium by their ability to contract in unison with other
smooth muscle cells. This is possible because of communicating junctions
between the cells constituting an electrical coupling of cells. Smooth muscle
cells lack transverse tubules, and their relatively small size allows them to

take up calcium ions from the matrix. They also have little sarcoplasmic reticulum. Smooth muscle cells have the ability to regenerate and are derived from mesoderm.

---

198. SUBJECT AREA: Muscle Tissue
QUESTION: Cardiac muscle cells

> *A:* are unique among the three types of muscle cells in that they lack intermediate filaments.
> *B:* in the atria are normally much larger in size than those in the ventricles.
> *C:* possess cell to cell junctions known as intercalated disks which are classified as desmosomes.
> *D:* can act as hormone secreting cells.
> *E:* are innervated by axons which terminate in end-plates similar to those of skeletal muscle.

Learning Response D: Correct. Cardiac myocytes in the atria are also hormone secreting cells and deliver atrial natriuretic protein to the blood stream. This hormone causes a sodium diuresis and a reduction in blood pressure. Atrial myocytes are smaller than their counterparts in the ventricles. Cardiac muscle cells possess intermediate filaments, some of which are associated in desmosomes which form a portion of a complex structure known as the intercalated disk. Small autonomic fibers innervate cardiac muscle and terminate in simplified synaptic contacts.

---

199. .SUBJECT AREA: Muscle Tissue
QUESTION: Actin in skeletal muscle cells

> *A:* is a highly conserved protein.
> *B:* has the ability to undergo transformations from a globular to a fibrous protein.
> *C:* forms the major protein component of the I bands.
> *D:* binds to troponin/tropomyosin as part of the calcium regulatory system of striated muscle.
> *E:* exhibits all of the above features.

Learning Response E: Correct. The amino acids sequence of actin from primitive eukaryotic cells is only slightly different from that of actin in mammalian muscle. Thus, it is a conserved protein with all of the features listed above.

---

200. SUBJECT AREA: Muscle Tissue

QUESTION: All of the following are characteristic of tropomyosin EXCEPT

A: its role as an actin binding protein.

B: its association with seven actin monomers in the thin filaments.

C: its location in the thin filaments of cardiac muscle.

D: the binding to troponin as part of the calcium regulatory system of striated muscle.

E: its requirement that it must be phosphorylated prior to binding actin.

Learning Response E: Correct. There is no requirement for the phosphorylation of tropomyosin for its binding to actin in the thin filaments.

---

201. SUBJECT AREA: Muscle Tissue

QUESTION: Satellite cells in skeletal muscle

A: constitute a population of undifferentiated cells.

B: are enclosed within the basal lamina of the skeletal muscle cells.

C: are activated by injury to the muscle.

D: are characterized by choices A, B and C above.

E: are characterized only by choices A and B above.

Learning Response D: Correct. Satellite cells within the basal lamina of skeletal muscle fibers provide an important role in the ability of skeletal muscle to regenerate after injury or trauma.

202. SUBJECT AREA: Muscle Tissue
   QUESTION: In skeletal muscle,

   A: myosin is dissociated from actin in the absence
       of ATP.
   B: the calcium binding proteins, calmodulin and
       troponin C, are associated with thin filaments.
   C: binding of acetylcholine to the sarcolemma makes
       the cell membrane more permeable to sodium ions.
   D: during sarcomere shortening, the I band shortens as
       a result of calcium-activated depolymerization of
       actin filaments.
   E: ATP released from the sarcoplasmic reticulum
       provides the energy for contraction.

Learning Response C: Correct. In the process of excitation-contraction coupling, acetylcholine receptors located in the sarcolemma bind to the neurotransmitter released from the axon terminal. This binding renders the cell membrane more permeable to sodium ions. Membrane depolarization is carried deep into the cell by the transverse tubules. In the absence of ATP produced by mitochondria, actin remains bound to myosin in the state of rigor. In smooth muscle, calmodulin binds calcium, activating the myosin light chain kinase prior to actomyosin interactions. Neither the I band nor the A band shortens during sarcomere shortening.

203. SUBJECT AREA: Muscle Tissue
   QUESTION: Intercalated disks of cardiac muscle can exhibit

   A: desmosomes.
   B: communicating or gap junctions.
   C: membrane specializations for the insertion of actin
       filaments.
   D: lateral and transverse regions.
   E: all of the above features.

Learning Response E: Correct. Cell to cell contacts between cardiac myocytes are specialized cell junctions known as intercalated disks. Their complex structure serves not only as anchoring junctions but also as areas of ion exchange between cells.

---

204. SUBJECT AREA: Muscle Tissue
QUESTION: Calcium regulation of smooth muscle cells

        A: requires the phosphorylation of myosin.
        B: is initiated by the binding of calcium
           by calmodulin.
        C: is mediated by activation of a myosin light
           chain kinase.
        D: involves choices A and B above.
        E: involves choices A, B and C above.

Learning Response E: Correct. Unlike calcium regulation of actin and myosin interactions in striated muscle, smooth muscle cells respond to calcium activation by the phosphorylation of myosin by a specific kinase, myosin light chain kinase. Calmodulin is the calcium binding protein.

---

205. SUBJECT AREA: Muscle Tissue
QUESTION: White skeletal muscle can be distinguished from red muscle by all of the following EXCEPT

        A: their content of myoglobin.
        B: their rate of contraction.
        C: the position of their nuclei.
        D: their source of energy.
        E: their numbers of mitochondria.

Learning Response C: Correct. Red and white muscles are two different classes of skeletal muscle, and both types have peripherally located nuclei. Red muscle has a higher content of myoglobin, contracts more slowly and has more mitochondria than white muscle. Red muscles derive their energy from oxidative phosphorylation while white muscle cells use anaerobic glycolysis.

206. SUBJECT AREA: Muscle Tissue

QUESTION: All of the following can be located in the A bands of striated muscle EXCEPT

    A: creatine kinase.
    B: actin.
    C: atriopeptin.
    D: tropomyosin.
    E: myosin.

Learning Response C: Correct. Atrial natriuretic factor or atriopeptin is localized in secretory granules in the sarcoplasm of cardiac muscle cells in the atria of the heart.

207. SUBJECT AREA: Muscle Tissue

QUESTION: Identify the structure indicated by the arrowheads in the figure below.

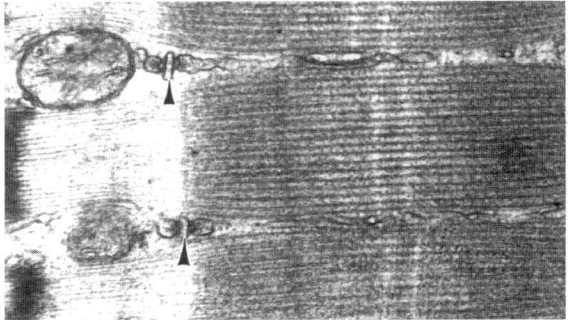

    A: thick filaments
    B: intermediate filaments
    C: thin filaments
    D: transverse tubules
    E: microtubules

Learning Response D: Correct. Transverse tubules are located at the lateral borders of the A bands in the sarcoplasm between the myofibrils of mammalian skeletal muscle. They convey the wave of membrane depolarization initiated at the neuromuscular junction deep into the cell.

208. SUBJECT AREA: Muscle Tissue
QUESTION: Identify the tissue depicted in the figure below.

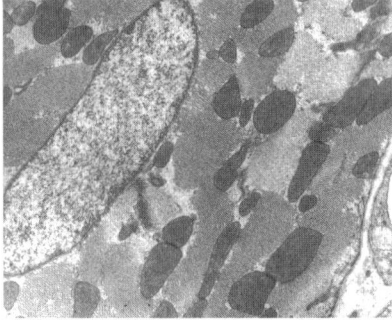

A: dense regular connective tissue
B: smooth muscle
C: cardiac muscle
D: loose connective tissue
E: skeletal muscle

Learning Response C: Correct. The central nucleus, abundant mitochondria and tranversely sectioned myofilaments indicate that this is a cardiac myocyte. The edge of the cell is located at the right of the image adjacent to a small blood vessel.

209. SUBJECT AREA: Muscle Tissue
QUESTION: Identify the tissue in the figure below.

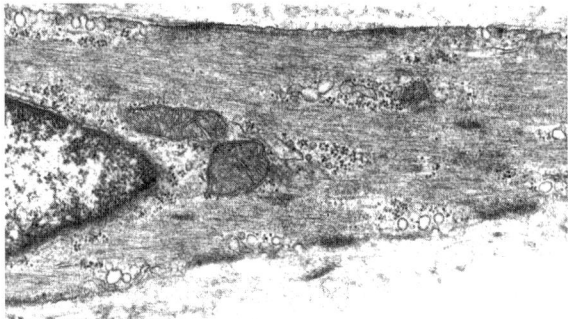

A: skeletal muscle
B: cardiac muscle
C: smooth muscle

> *D:* dense connective tissue
> *E:* nerve

Learning Response C: Correct. The shape of the cell, the centrally located nucleus and the little extracellular material are clues in identifying this as smooth muscle. Cardiac muscle cells are striated. Skeletal muscle nuclei are peripherally distributed. The delicate connective tissue fibers indicate that this is not dense connective tissue, and the paucity of rough endoplasmic reticulum suggests that this is not a nerve cell.

---

210. SUBJECT AREA: Muscle Tissue
    QUESTION: Identify the specific region of the sarcomere in which the arrowhead is located in the figure below.

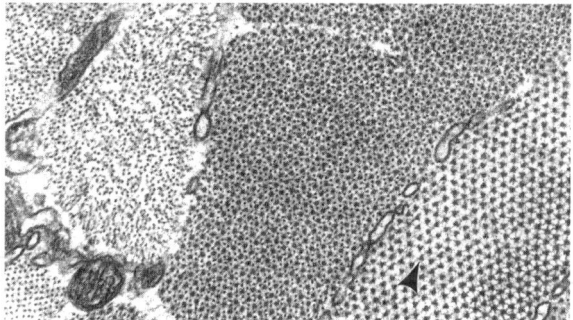

> *A:* I band
> *B:* Z line
> *C:* H zone
> *D:* M line
> *E:* A band

Learning Response C: Correct. The tip of the arrowhead points to a thick filament which is not surrounded by thin filaments such as those to the left of the arrowhead. In addition, there are no connections between the thick filaments such as those to the right of the arrowhead. The I band containing only thin filaments is located at the left edge of the image, and the Z line in the lower left corner. Response E, A band, would technically be correct since the H zone is part of the A band.

211. SUBJECT AREA: Muscle Tissue
QUESTION: Identify the tissue shown in the figure below.

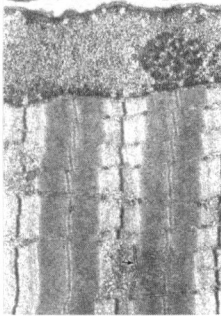

A: smooth muscle
B: cardiac muscle
C: nerve
D: skeletal muscle
E: dense connective tissue

Learning Response D: Correct. The presence of cross striations and the peripherally located nucleus confirm that this is a section through skeletal muscle. Note the elongated T-tubule in the lower center of the field (arrow).

212. SUBJECT AREA: Muscle Tissue
QUESTION: In the figure below, identify the structure marked by the arrowhead.

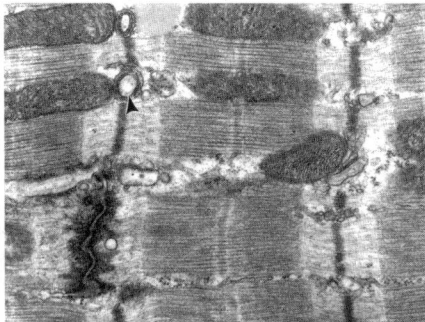

A: sarcoplasmic reticulum
B: lipid

C: mitochondrion
D: intercalated disk
E: tranverse tubule

Learning Response E: Correct. In this longitudinal section through a cardiac muscle cell, the transverse tubules (T-tubules) are located in the sarcoplasm at the level of the Z line. In mammalian skeletal muscle, T-tubules can be found at the lateral borders of the A bands. An intercalated disk can be seen at the lower left of the field.

213. SUBJECT AREA Muscle Tissue

QUESTION When actin thin filaments that are attached to the Z line in striated muscle are decorated with heavy meromyosin, the barbed or plus end of the filaments faces the

A: Z line.
B: M line.
C: A band.
D: H zone.
E: I band.

Learning Response A: Correct. The barbed end of decorated thin filaments faces the Z line, and the pointed end is directed toward the A band, H zone, M line. Thus, the thin filaments exhibit a polarity of structure. The plus end of the filaments is that region where actin monomers are preferentially added.

214. SUBJECT AREA Muscle Tissue

QUESTION In smooth muscle, the binding of calcium to calmodulin ultimately can result in

A: activation of myosin light chain kinase.
B: phosphorylation of myosin light polypeptide chains.
C: activation of myosin ATPase.
D: formation of myosin filaments.
E: all of the above events.

Learning Response E: Correct. Regulation of smooth muscle myosin and actin interactions by calcium produces at some time or another all the events listed above.

215. SUBJECT AREA: Nervous System

QUESTION: When a neuron dies, those neurons with which it synapses remain functionally intact except in the case where there is only one link. This neuron, once isolated, undergoes

A: chromatolysis.
B: transneuronal degeneration.
C: saltatory conduction.
D: antidromic spread.
E: gliosis.

Learning Response B: Correct. Chromatolysis is common to all dying neurons, but transneuronal degeneration is specific to isolated neurons. Saltatory conduction and antidromic spread refer to the propagation of the action potential along myelinated nerve fibers and the diffusion of the wave of depolarization toward the cell body, respectively. Gliosis is the result of astrocyte proliferation after nerve injury.

216. SUBJECT AREA: Nervous System

QUESTION: Just as the Schwann cell produces the myelin sheath for neurons in the peripheral nervous system (PNS), central nervous system (CNS) neurons are myelinated by

A: oligodendrocytes.
B: microglia.
C: astrocytes.
D: satellite cells.
E: none of the above; all CNS neurons are unmyelinated.

Learning Response A: Correct. In contrast to their counterparts in the peripheral nervous system, the Schwann cells which myelinate only one axon, oligodendrocytes in the CNS can myelinate up to 50 axons. Microglia are macrophages; astrocytes provide structural and trophic support. Satellite cells surround ganglia in the PNS. Some CNS neurons are unmyelinated, but not all.

---

217. SUBJECT AREA: Nervous System
QUESTION: Axon terminals contain

> *A:* Golgi complex.
> *B:* postsynaptic receptors.
> *C:* Nissl substance.
> *D:* autoreceptors.
> *E:* initial segments.

Learning Response D: Correct. Postsynaptic receptors can be found on the shaft of the recipient axon in axoaxonic synapses, but there are no axo-terminaux bouton synapses (no afferent synapses directly on the axon terminal itself). Autoreceptors are an important feedback mechanism by which the neurotransmitter at the axon terminal can inhibit further release.

---

218. SUBJECT AREA: Nervous System
QUESTION: The following are all characteristics of a dendrite EXCEPT

> *A:* arborization.
> *B:* Nissl substance.
> *C:* varying diameter with continued branching.
> *D:* initial segment.
> *E:* postsynaptic receptors.

Learning Response D: Correct. The initial segment is the site on an axon of multiple ion channels (both inhibitory and excitatory) resulting in the initiation of propagation of the action potential in myelinated neurons.

---

219. SUBJECT AREA: Nervous System
QUESTION: An axon

A: can synapse directly with another neuron only through dendrites.

B: must be surrounded by layers of myelin to propagate an action potential.

C: occasionally has collateral branches.

D: cannot regenerate past the initial site of injury.

E: receives only excitatory input.

Learning Response C: Correct. An axon also can synapse with the cell body (axosomatic) or another axon (axoaxonic) and can receive both excitatory and inhibitory inputs. Unmyelinated nerve fibers can also generate action potentials.

220. SUBJECT AREA: Nervous System

QUESTION: All of the following are components of the blood-brain barrier EXCEPT

A: occluding junctions.

B: minimal pinocytotic vesicles.

C: fenestrated endothelium with thin diaphragms.

D: astrocytic foot processes.

E: endothelial cell basal lamina.

Learning Response C: Correct. Fenestrated endothelium is not found in the blood vessels supplying the brain. In addition, research has demonstrated that astrocytes are a major component of the blood-brain barrier and can alter the structure of the endothelial cell membrane, thereby making it impermeable.

221. SUBJECT AREA: Nervous System

QUESTION: The autonomic nervous system

A: is located entirely within the peripheral nervous system.

B: is involved only in maintaining homeostasis.

C: is involved only in "fight-or-flight" responses.

D: has both motor and sensory components.

E: is primarily composed of bipolar neurons.

Learning Response D: Correct. The parasympathetic component of the autonomic nervous system has nuclei within the midbrain and medulla of the brain. Autonomic neurons are usually multipolar; bipolar neurons are rare.

---

222. SUBJECT AREA: Nervous System
QUESTION: Axonal transport

> *A:* is the propagation of the stimulatory input down to the axon terminal.
> *B:* relies on elements of the axonal cytoskeleton.
> *C:* is unidirectional.
> *D:* involves mobilization of Nissl substance into the perikaryon.
> *E:* is the propagation of inhibitory input back to the neuronal cell body.

Learning Response B: Correct. The flow of cytoplasmic components (proteins, mitochondria, vesicles, etc.) within the axon is bidirectional. The neuronal cytoskeleton including microtubules and microfilaments is involved in axonal transport. Agents which disrupt microtubules and microfilaments slow axonal transport.

---

223. SUBJECT AREA: Nervous System
QUESTION: Neuronal regeneration and reinnervation

> *A:* does not occur in the central nervous system (CNS).
> *B:* is entirely dependent on vascularization.
> *C:* occurs only with sensory neurons, not motor neurons.
> *D:* can only occur in myelinated neurons.
> *E:* is dependent on both glial cells and the target tissue.

Learning Response E: Correct. Oligodendrocytes in the CNS, Schwann cells in the PNS, and target tissue growth factors are essential in regeneration/reinnervation to supply both trophic support and axonal guidance.

224. SUBJECT AREA: Nervous System
QUESTION: The lining of the choroid plexus is

A: ciliated cuboidal epithelium.
B: unfenestrated endothelium.
C: pseudostratified, ciliated columnar epithelium.
D: unciliated simple columnar epithelium.
E: columnar epithelium with microvilli.

Learning Response E: Correct. The ependyma elsewhere in the brain has ciliated cuboidal epithelium, but the specialized lining of the choroid plexus is columnar with microvilli.

225. SUBJECT AREA: Nervous System
QUESTION: All of the following are components of the blood-cerebrospinal fluid (CSF) barrier EXCEPT

A: astrocytic foot processes.
B: fenestrated capillaries with diaphragms.
C: tight junctions in the endothelium.
D: epithelial cell basement membrane.
E: endothelial cell basement membrane.

Learning Response A: Correct. The astrocytic foot processes (also known as the glia limitans or glial limiting membrane) is a major component of the blood-brain barrier, not the blood-CSF barrier. The endothelial cells (pia mater capillaries) and epithelial cells (continuations of the ependyma) form this barrier. These specialized ependymal cells do have a basement membrane.

226. SUBJECT AREA: Nervous System
QUESTION: A component common to both autonomic and dorsal root ganglia (DRG) is

A: pseudounipolar neurons.
B: satellite cells.
C: motor and receptive functions.

D: normal dendritic tree expansion from
the perikaryon.
E: parasympathetic input.

Learning Response B: Correct. Autonomic neurons are usually multipolar, whereas DRG neurons are pseudounipolar. DRGs are only sensory, receiving input from the distal axon, not a dendritic tree. Satellite cells contribute to the support of neurons in both types of ganglia.

227. SUBJECT AREA: Nervous System
QUESTION: In regard to the linings of the brain, all of the following are true EXCEPT

A: all the meninges are found on both the external and internal surfaces of the brain.
B: the dura is continuous with the periosteum.
C: the arachnoid is continuous with the ventricles.
D: the pia mater is not in direct contact with neurons.
E: the pia does not surround capillaries in the central nervous system.

Learning Response A: Correct. The meninges are only found on the external surface of the brain; the ependyma lines the internal surface (ventricles). Even at the choroid plexus and arachnoid granulations, specialized ependymal cells (not a meningeal layer) line the lumenal surface.

228. SUBJECT AREA: Nervous System
QUESTION: When a neuron is at resting potential,

A: the intracellular calcium concentration is 20 times lower than the extracellular concentration.
B: sodium ions are ten times more concentrated on the inside of the neuron than on the outside.
C: there is no net movement of potassium ions.
D: the interior of the neuron is 40-100 mV more positive than the exterior.

> *E:* the intracellular potassium concentration is much lower than the extracellular concentration.

Learning Response C: Correct. At resting potential, the inside of the neuron is much more negative (due to high potassium ion concentration) than the outside (due to high sodium ion concentration).

---

229. SUBJECT AREA: Nervous System
QUESTION: In generating an axon potential due to excitatory synaptic input, all of the following are true EXCEPT

> *A:* the presynaptic vesicles usually contain the neurotransmitter GABA (gamma-aminobutyric acid).
> *B:* the initial segment of the axon is involved.
> *C:* sodium channels open.
> *D:* orthodromic spread depolarizes adjacent regions of the membrane.
> *E:* potassium channels stay open for a longer time than sodium channels.

Learning Response A: Correct. GABA neurons are inhibitory, not excitatory.

---

230. SUBJECT AREA: Nervous System
QUESTION: All of the following are functions of myelin EXCEPT

> *A:* maintenance of a low capacitance of the axonal membrane.
> *B:* the rapid, passive spread of the depolarization current along the membrane.
> *C:* insulation of the axon from further synaptic input.
> *D:* to provide trophic support to the axon.
> *E:* reduction in the energy required for ion pumps.

Learning Response D: Correct. There is no evidence that myelin itself is trophic for an axon. An axon receives its trophic support from the neuronal cell body and from glial cells.

231. SUBJECT AREA: Nervous System

QUESTION: In an electron micrograph, synaptic function can be determined sometimes by all of the following characteristics of the synaptic vesicles EXCEPT

A: size.
B: electron opacity of the contents.
C: shape.
D: proximity to the initial segment.
E: presence of a dense core surrounded by a clear area.

Learning Response D: Correct. Those synapses at the initial segment are the most influential inputs, but can have either an excitatory or inhibitory function.

232. SUBJECT AREA: Nervous System

QUESTION: Components of the parasympathetic nervous system

A: are primarily located within the thoracolumbar region.
B: secrete norepinephrine.
C: have short preganglionic fibers.
D: include the vagus nerve.
E: have a less discrete, more generalized effect than the sympathetic system.

Learning Response D: Correct. Since the parasympathetic neurotransmitter (acetylcholine) is degraded more rapidly in the synapse than the sympathetic transmitter (norepinephrine) is degraded by monoamine oxidases, it has a more discrete and localized action.

233. SUBJECT AREA: Nervous System

QUESTION: The effect of the synaptic input to a neuron can be influenced by all of the following EXCEPT

A: width of the postsynaptic membrane.

B: number of inhibitory inputs.
C: number of excitatory inputs.
D: location of the input at the initial segment.
E: location of the input at a dendritic spine.

Learning Response A: Correct. There is no evidence of a correlation between postsynaptic density and synaptic effect. The most influential factor is the location of the input (excitatory or inhibitory) to the initial segment where the majority of ion-gated channels are located and the action potential is propagated initially.

234. SUBJECT AREA: Nervous System
       QUESTION: At the node of Ranvier

A: sodium and potassium channels are concentrated.
B: saltatory conduction is terminated.
C: the endoneurium intervenes between the Schwann cell and the axon.
D: voltage-gated channels are closed or inactivated.
E: calcium channels are concentrated.

Learning Response A: Correct. Conduction of depolarization from one node to the next (saltatory conduction) occurs at the nodes by activation of the voltage-gated channels concentrated there. Calcium channels, at the axon terminal, are involved in the fusion of secretory vesicles with the presynaptic membrane and exocytosis.

235. SUBJECT AREA: Nervous System
       QUESTION: Cerebrospinal fluid (CSF)

A: has a composition similar to blood.
B: is produced by arachnoid granulations.
C: fills the extensive extracellular spaces within the central nervous system.
D: serves both a metabolic and protective function.
E: is recirculated via lymphatic channels.

Learning Response D: Correct. CSF (produced by the choroid plexus and absorbed at the arachnoid granulations) has an ionic composition similar to plasma, but has a low density, very low protein content and very few cells. There are no lymphatic vessels in the brain.

---

236. SUBJECT AREA: Nervous System
QUESTION: White matter is composed primarily of all of the following EXCEPT

   A: axons.
   B: oligodendrocytes.
   C: perikarya.
   D: fibrous astrocytes.
   E: microglia.

Learning Response C: Correct. Perikarya (neuronal cell bodies) are located in nuclei and gray matter.

---

237. SUBJECT AREA: Nervous System
QUESTION: Several human demyelinating diseases are due to an insufficiency in, or lack of,

   A: oligodendrocytes.
   B: mesaxons.
   C: Schwann cells.
   D: microglia.
   E: myelin basic protein (MBP).

Learning Response E: Correct. MBP and proteolipid protein are major components of myelin. In some demyelinating diseases, the glial cell functions normally but an immune reaction to the MBP results in the destruction of the myelin itself.

---

238. SUBJECT AREA: Nervous System
QUESTION: All of the following occur at a cholinergic synapse EXCEPT

> *A:* choline is transported into the terminal with
> a sodium gradient.
> *B:* choline acetyltransferase combines free choline
> with acetate.
> *C:* voltage-sensitive calcium channels open.
> *D:* only postsynaptic receptors bind the released
> acetylcholine.
> *E:* acetylcholinesterase degrades excess acetylcholine
> within the synaptic cleft.

Learning Response D: Correct. Many cholinergic neurons have presynaptic receptors for acetylcholine. These autoreceptors are a major feedback mechanism by which the further release of neurotransmitter is inhibited.

239. SUBJECT AREA: Nervous System
QUESTION: At the synapse,

> *A:* vesicles are released and taken up by the
> postsynaptic neuron.
> *B:* microglial foot processes block diffusion of
> neurotransmitters away from the synaptic cleft.
> *C:* saltatory conduction is propagated.
> *D:* the synaptic web or density is on the postsynaptic
> side of the synaptic cleft.
> *E:* only one neurotransmitter is released at a time.

Learning Response D: Correct. Only the contents of the vesicles, not the vesicles themselves, are released. A number of neurotransmitters are co-localized within the same vesicles (e.g. acetylcholine and VIP).

240. SUBJECT AREA: Nervous System
QUESTION: The sympathetic nervous system can be identified by
all of the following EXCEPT

> *A:* short preganglionic fibers.
> *B:* norepinephrine neurotransmission.
> *C:* splanchnic nerves.

D: thoracic location.

E: intramural ganglia located within effector organs.

Learning Response E: Correct. The parasympathetic system has intramural ganglia within the walls of the target organs.

241. SUBJECT AREA: Nervous System

QUESTION: When a nerve fiber is damaged in the central nervous system,

A: the distal end can be metabolically supported by oligodendrocytes until the proximal end regrows.

B: the perikaryon also dies.

C: microglia are active in the removal of the debris.

D: fibrous astrocytes maintain an open pathway for the sprouting axon.

E: the target neuron has no effect on regeneration or reinnervation.

Learning Response C: Correct. Oligodendrocytes can maintain an open pathway for reinnervation, but do not metabolically support the distal end. Trophic factors secreted by the target neuron maintain the afferent neuron and signal the correct pathway for reinnervation.

242. SUBJECT AREA: Nervous System

QUESTION: All of the following are true about glial cells EXCEPT that they

A: contain receptors for certain neurotransmitters.

B: are all found in both white and gray matter.

C: are a component of all synaptic junctions.

D: contain some neuropeptides.

E: may damage neurons, as well as support them.

Learning Response C: Correct. In certain diseases (e.g., Alzheimer's, perhaps AIDS-related complex), some of the compounds secreted by glia (e.g., nitrous oxide, cytokines) are toxic to neurons.

243. SUBJECT AREA: Nervous System
QUESTION: Unmyelinated axons

> A: are not found in the peripheral nervous system.
> B: need nodes of Ranvier for propagation of action potentials.
> C: have a slow conduction velocity.
> D: have such a large diameter that a Schwann cell cannot completely ensheath them.
> E: cannot regenerate due to the lack of glial guidance.

Learning Response C: Correct. Unmyelinated axons in both the peripheral and central nervous systems usually are covered by a layer of glia; they just are not fully wrapped with multiple layers of myelin. In addition, axons without any glial sheath do exist in the CNS; these regenerate with the help of adjacent glia.

244. SUBJECT AREA: Nervous System
QUESTION: At a noradrenergic synapse,

> A: calcium influx potentiates the fusion of synaptic vesicles with the presynaptic membrane.
> B: dopamine β-hydroxylase converts epinephrine to norepinephrine.
> C: tyrosine cannot be taken up on the presynaptic side.
> D: cocaine augments the reuptake of norepinephrine.
> E: monoamine oxidase (MAO) causes the formation of more norepinephrine.

Learning Response A: Correct. Cocaine blocks the reuptake of norepinephrine (NE), thereby removing the inhibition of continued secretion from the presynaptic terminal and, effectively, acting as a stimulus for continued NE secretion. In contrast, MAOs enzymatically inactivate NE.

245. SUBJECT AREA: Nervous System
QUESTION: Dorsal root ganglia (DRG)

A: are a component of the sympathetic nervous system.

B: have satellite cells.

C: contain multipolar neurons.

D: contain interneurons for continued impulse conduction.

E: usually convey motor information.

Learning Response B: Correct. DRGs (spinal or sensory ganglia) contain pseudounipolar neurons that conduct sensory information; they synapse with interneurons inside the spinal cord, not in the ganglion itself.

---

246. SUBJECT AREA: Nervous System

QUESTION: Oligodendrocytes

A: are the most prominent glial cell in gray matter.

B: have perivascular end-feet.

C: are of mesenchymal/mesodermal origin.

D: have a metabolic interdependency with neurons.

E: are involved in maintaining the blood-brain barrier.

Learning Response D: Correct. Astrocytes are the most prominent glial cell type: fibrous astrocytes provide structural support; the perivascular end-feet of protoplasmic astrocytes are components of the blood-brain barrier. Microglia are mesodermally derived cells of macrophage/monocyte lineage.

---

247. SUBJECT AREA: Nervous System

QUESTION: In the spinal cord,

A: there is no arachnoid layer between the dura and pia.

B: input from pseudounipolar neurons enters the dorsal horns.

C: there are no interneurons.

D: the small perikarya making up the majority of the anterior horn population have a sensory modality.

E: ascending fibers do not cross to the contralateral side.

Learning Response B: Correct. The spinal cord is the best place to visualize the arachnoid layer, grossly and histologically. Ventral horn cells are large cells and function as motor neurons.

---

248. SUBJECT AREA: Nervous System
QUESTION: In the cerebellum,

> *A:* the molecular layer of the cortex is primarily unmyelinated fibers.
> *B:* Purkinje cells are located between the internal layer of white matter and the granule cells.
> *C:* granule cells are primarily found within the vermis.
> *D:* granule layer neurons are larger than the perikarya of the molecular layer.
> *E:* Purkinje cells are the smallest neurons in the brain.

Learning Response A: Correct. In between the two layers of cerebellar gray matter (outer molecular layer and inner granular cell layer) are the largest cells in the brain, the Purkinje cells. In the cerebellum, the gray matter is the outer or surface layer and white matter is the internal layer.

---

249. SUBJECT AREA: Nervous System
QUESTION: During development of the nervous system,

> *A:* the neural crest gives rise to the neural groove.
> *B:* pseudounipolar neurons are formed by the fusion of two processes of a multipolar neuron.
> *C:* trophic factors often are secreted by the target organ to guide the direction of axonal growth.
> *D:* only neuronal structures are derived from the neural crest.
> *E:* satellite cells are mesodermally derived.

Learning Response C: Correct. This is a critical concept in neuronal plasticity and survival. Neural crest cells are located lateral to the neural groove and form the neurons and support cells of the peripheral nervous system and the neurons that constitute the diffuse neuroendocrine system.

250. SUBJECT AREA: Nervous System
QUESTION: The ependymal lining of the ventricular surfaces of the brain is different from most epithelia because it

A: lacks a basal lamina.
B: is mesodermally derived.
C: contains few occluding junctions.
D: serves a trophic function.
E: has cilia.

Learning Response A: Correct. Not all epithelia have tight junctions (e.g., renal tubules, glandular epithelia), but they all have a basal lamina. Ependymal cells are an exception to this generality.

251. SUBJECT AREA: Nervous System
QUESTION: In the central nervous system,

A: lymphocytes readily cross the blood-brain barrier.
B: lymphocytes readily cross the blood-ependymal barrier.
C: microglial cells are the only endogenous immunocytes.
D: lymphatic drainage occurs at the sites where the blood-brain barrier is leaky.
E: neurons are impervious to cytokine stimulation.

Learning Response C: Correct. There is a slight amount of lymphocyte trafficking into the brain normally, but it accounts for a very minor component of the endogenous immunocyte population. Research has demonstrated unequivocally that neurons in many regions of the brain (especially the hypothalamic neuroendocrine neurons) are responsive to both endogenous (produced by microglia and astrocytes) and systemic cytokines.

252. SUBJECT AREA: Nervous System
QUESTION: A peripheral nerve is composed of all of the following EXCEPT

A: perineurial fibroblasts.

> *B:* many axons conducting motor and sensory
>   modalities.
> *C:* Schwann cells.
> *D:* lymphatic vessels.
> *E:* endoneurial reticular fibers.

Learning Response D: Correct. Lymphatic vessels are not present in
nervous tissue.

253. SUBJECT AREA: Nervous System
> QUESTION: Some of the largest cells in the body are in the nervous
>   system. Which of the following does NOT belong in
>   this group?

> *A:* cerebellar Purkinje cells
> *B:* spinal motor neurons
> *C:* sensory ganglion neurons
> *D:* cerebellar granular neurons
> *E:* sympathetic ganglion cells

Learning Response D: Correct. Cerebellar granular neurons, approximately
the size of erythrocytes, are among the smallest cells in the body.

254. SUBJECT AREA: Nervous System
> QUESTION: At the neuromuscular junction of skeletal muscle,

> *A:* the sarcoplasmic membrane contains receptors for
>   acetylcholine.
> *B:* there is no Schwann cell.
> *C:* the axon terminal contains junctional folds.
> *D:* satellite cells contain acetylcholine esterase.
> *E:* one axon commonly innervates only one
>   muscle fiber.

Learning Response A: Correct. The axon loses its myelin sheath, but the
Schwann cell still provides a thin cytoplasmic covering over the area of the
axon terminal not in contact with the muscle cell membrane. The muscle fiber

exhibits folds at the surface closest to the axon. Acetylcholine is degraded by enzemes in the cleft between the axon and muscle cell.Only movements requiring a fine degree of control, such as those of the extraocular muscles usually result in a 1:1 axon to muscle cell ratio.

255. SUBJECT AREA: Nervous System

QUESTION: The major neurotransmitter of the parasympathetic nervous system is

A: acetylcholine.
B: norepinephrine.
C: epinephrine.
D: choline.
E: GABA.

Learning Response A: Correct. Choline itself is not a transmitter. Acetylcholine is rapidly broken down by esterases, and therefore, the innervation is more localized and of finite duration.

256. SUBJECT AREA: Nervous System

QUESTION: Identify the nucleated cell depicted in the figure below?

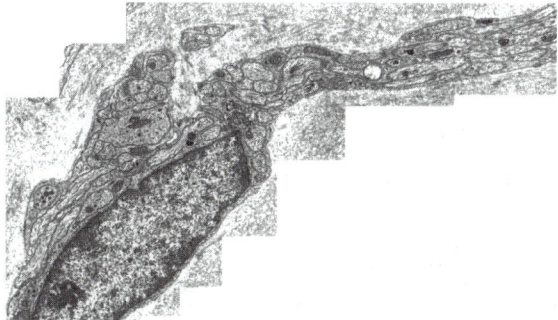

A: oligodendrocyte
B: astrocyte
C: Schwann cell
D: satellite
E: microglial cell

Learning Response C: Correct. The nucleated cell is a Schwann cell located in the peripheral nervous system. Its cytoplasm surrounds several unmyelinated axons. Oligodendrocytes, astrocytes and microglia are all found in the central nervous system. Satellite cells provide support for neurons in ganglia.

---

257. SUBJECT AREA: Nervous System

QUESTION: The photomicrograph in the figure below shows structures in the dermis of skin that

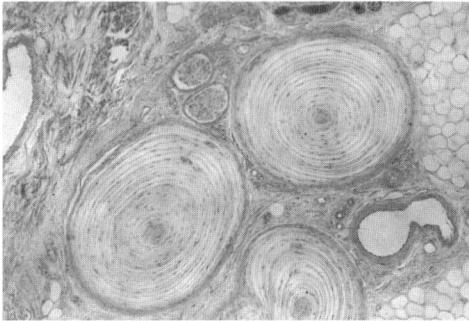

A: are intramural parasympathetic ganglia.

B: contain somatic efferent neurons.

C: are chemoreceptors.

D: contain the distal axon of a pseudounipolar neuron from a dorsal root ganglion.

E: convey sensory modality to the paravertebral sympathetic ganglia.

Learning Response D: Correct. Pacinian corpuscles are mechanoreceptors for vibration or deep pressure and are the most distal portion of a pseudounipolar axon which has its cell body in a dorsal root ganglion.

---

258. SUBJECT AREA: Nervous System

QUESTION: All of the following are released from neuroendocrine synapses EXCEPT

A: CCK-8 (cholecystokinin 1-8).

B: VIP (vasoactive intestinal peptide).

C: somatostatin.

D: serotonin (5-hydroxytryptamine).
E: secretin.

Learning Response E: Correct. All these hormones of the diffuse neuroendocrine system were originally isolated and characterized from the gut, hence the gut-related names. However, the same compound has also been shown to be synthesized and released within the brain.

259. SUBJECT AREA: Nervous System
QUESTION: When an axon is injured, the trauma is reflected in the cell body or perikaryon by

    A: axoplasmic transport.
    B: the release of neurotransmitter.
    C: demyelination.
    D: chromatolysis, a dissolution of Nissl substance.
    E: enhanced axon potentials.

Learning Response D: Correct. Axonal injury results in the dissolution of Nissl substance, an increase in volume of the perikaryon and the migration of the nucleus to the periphery of the perikaryon.

260. SUBJECT AREA: Nervous System
QUESTION: Myelin has all of the following features EXCEPT that

    A: its sheaths are formed by the juxtaposition of the plasma membrane layers of Schwann cells.
    B: its sheaths are interrupted by nodes of Ranvier.
    C: it surrounds all but the smallest axons.
    D: it has no effect on the speed of impulse conduction.
    E: it is present in both the central and peripheral nervous systems.

Learning Response D: Correct. Myelination increases the speed of conduction of the action potential. The nerve impulse travels rapidly from node to node, a process called saltatory conduction.

261. SUBJECT AREA: Nervous System
QUESTION: Neuroglia

> *A:* help control the chemical and electrical environment of neurons.
> *B:* are unipolar cells.
> *C:* are required only in the mature nervous system.
> *D:* remain postmitotic throughout the adult life of an individual.
> *E:* have cell bodies which are the same size as most neuronal cell bodies.

Learning Response A: Correct. Neuroglia have receptors for neurotransmitters and synthesize peptides that are also common to neurons, and can produce trophic or toxic substances.

262. .SUBJECT AREA: Nervous System
QUESTION: All of the following are features of the perineurium EXCEPT

> *A:* for its composition of flattened epithelial-like cells.
> *B:* for the presence of tight junctions between its cellular components.
> *C:* that it can act as a barrier isolating nerve fibers beneath it from macromolecules.
> *D:* that it fills in the spaces between nerve fiber bundles, analogous to perimysium of skeletal muscle.
> *E:* that it stains darker than the epineurium in histological sections.

Learning Response D: Correct. The perineurium functions differently from perimysium which fills in the spaces between bundles of skeletal muscle fibers. In nerve fibers, epineurium is the dense connective tissue which is located between bundles of nerve fibers.

263. SUBJECT AREA: Nervous System
QUESTION: Dendrites have all of the following structures EXCEPT

A: neurofilaments.
B: Golgi complex.
C: microtubules.
D: Nissl substance.
E: mitochondria.

Learning Response B: Correct. Dendrites and axons have a number of structures in common, such as microtubules, neurofilaments and mitochondria. Nissl substance is found in the neuronal cell body and in dendrites, not in axons. Neither dendrites nor axons have any of the elements of the Golgi complex.

264. SUBJECT AREA: Nervous System
QUESTION: The major dense lines of the myelin sheath

A: represent the fused outer surfaces of the Schwann cell plasma membrane.
B: consist of compressed bundles of microfilaments in the Schwann cell.
C: represent the fused cytoplasmic surfaces of the Schwann cell plasma membrane.
D: represent axonal cytoplasm compressed by the Schwann cell.
E: would be absent from myelinated axons in the central nervous system.

Learning Response C: Correct. As the Schwann cell wraps around the axon, its cytoplasm is compressed against the inner lipid layer of its plasma membrane resulting in the formation of the major dense line. The intraperiod line represents the fused outer surfaces of the Schwann cell membrane.

265. SUBJECT AREA: Circulatory System
QUESTION: The lymphatic system

A: returns interstitial fluid to the circulation.
B: begins in blind-ended capillaries.
C: plays an important role in the immune response.
D: contains lymphatic capillaries which are not fenestrated.

E: is characterized by all of the above.

Learning Response E: Correct. The lymphatic system is responsible for returning interstitial fluid to the general circulation. It begins as blind-ended lymphatic capillaries, which are lined by a single layer of nonfenestrated endothelial cells. These channels converge to form larger lymphatic vessels which resemble veins in that valves are present. However, lymph vessels have thinner walls as compared to veins of similar size; it is also harder to distinguish the three tunics in lymph vessels. The larger lymphatic vessels ultimately form two large lymphatic ducts which, like veins, contain smooth muscle in the media. The lymphatic ducts empty in the venous system, thereby returning the fluid to the circulation. Interposed along the course of the lymphatic vessels are lymph nodes which function in immune responses.

266. SUBJECT AREA: Circulatory System
QUESTION: The tunica intima

A: has a subendothelial layer of loose connective tissue and occasional smooth muscle.
B: is separated from the tunica media by the internal elastic lamina (in arteries).
C: contains cells which line the vessel's interior surface.
D: contains cells which are metabolically active.
E: is characterized by all of the above.

Learning Response E: Correct. Blood vessels contain three layers, or tunics, the innermost of which is the tunica intima composed of endothelial which line the vessel's interior surface. Endothelial cells perform a variety of functions, including conversion of angiotensin I to angiotensin II and conversion of bradykinin, norepinephrine, and other substances to inert compounds. In addition, endothelial cells serve an antithrombogenic function in that they separate blood platelets from the highly thrombogenic subendothelial connective tissue. This subendothelial layer of connective tissue is included in the tunica intima and is separated from the smooth muscle of the underlying tunica media by the internal elastic lamina.

267. SUBJECT AREA: Circulatory System
QUESTION: An elderly patient is afflicted with abnormalities of the right leg. The physician determines that this is the result of arterial insufficiency secondary to compression of the right femoral artery by an angiosarcoma (malignant tumor of blood vessels). The cell that is most likely responsible for this is a(n)

    A: Purkinje cell.
    B: endothelial cell.
    C: red blood cell.
    D: fibroblast.
    E: cardiac myocyte.

Learning Response B: Correct. The majority of malignant tumors of blood vessels are derived from endothelial cells or pericytes.

268. Subject Area: Circulatory System
QUESTION: Which of the following associations is NOT correct?

    A: somatic capillaries—muscle tissue
    B: fenestrated capillaries with diaphragms—intestine, endocrine glands
    C: sinusoidal capillaries—nerve tissue
    D: fenestrated capillaries without diaphragms—renal glomerulus
    E: sinusoidal capillaries—discontinuous basal lamina

Learning Response C: Correct. There are four types of capillaries. Type I is the continuous (somatic) capillary found in muscle tissue, connective tissue, exocrine glands, and nervous tissue. Endothelial cells of these capillaries are not fenestrated. Type II is the fenestrated (visceral) capillary of the kidney, intestine, and endocrine glands. The fenestrae are covered by a thin diaphragm and a continuous basal lamina is present. Type III is unique to the renal glomerulus and is also a fenestrated capillary, but the fenestrae are not covered by diaphragms. A thick basal lamina is present. Type IV is the sinusoidal capillary of the liver, bone marrow, and spleen. The endothelial cells are fenestrated (with diaphragms) and the basal lamina is discontinuous.

269. SUBJECT AREA: Circulatory System
QUESTION: Which of the following associations is NOT correct?

 A: pulmonary arteries—thinner walls as compared to renal arteries
 B: capillaries—tunica media composed of pericytes
 C: large veins of the abdomen and legs—smooth muscle in the adventitia
 D: capillaries—no tunica adventitia
 E: venules—thin walls as compared to an artery of the same diameter

Learning Response D: Correct. Blood vessels contain three layers, although they may be more or less developed depending on the given vessel. Thus, in a capillary the tunica intima is composed of endothelial cells, the tunica media is composed of pericytes, and the tunica adventitia is composed of a thin layer of surrounding reticular fibers. One should also remember various structural modifications: the walls of arteries are thicker than that of similarly sized veins, large veins of the abdomen and extremities contain abundant smooth muscle in the adventitia to assist blood return to the heart; the pulmonary circulation has a lower pressure, and, therefore, its vessels have thinner walls as compared to the systemic arteries.

270. SUBJECT AREA: Circulatory System
QUESTION: In reference to capillaries and metarterioles,

 A: the precapillary sphincter is composed of skeletal muscle.
 B: metarterioles maintain pressure differences within the circulatory system.
 C: in contrast to skeletal muscle, smooth muscle is likely to have a well developed capillary network.
 D: constriction of metarterioles may completely stop blood flow within capillaries.
 E: all of the above statements are correct.

Learning Response B: Correct. Metarterioles contain a discontinuous layer of smooth muscle, constriction of which allows these vessels to maintain pressure differences between the arterial and venous systems. However, only constriction of the precapillary sphincter, a simple ring of smooth muscle at the site of capillary origin, can completely stop blood flow through a given capillary. The abundance of the capillary network in a tissue is related to its metabolic activity. Thus, active tissues such as skeletal muscle, liver, and kidney are likely to have more capillaries than less active tissues such as dense connective tissue.

271. SUBJECT AREA: Circulatory System
QUESTION: A deficiency in the protein contained in Weibel-Palade granules would result in

  A: a type of connective tissue disorder.
  B: a type of immune deficiency.
  C: increased platelet adhesion to injured endothelium.
  D: a type of hemophilia.
  E: none of the above conditions.

Learning Response D: Correct. Weibel-Palade granules are found in endothelial cells of vessels larger than capillaries and contain a protein known as von Willebrand's factor (factor VIII). This protein plays a vital role in the coagulation cascade; therefore, a deficiency causes a type of hemophilia. In von Willebrand's disease, the loss of this factor leads to decreased platelet adhesion to injured endothelium and prolonged bleeding time.

272. SUBJECT AREA: Circulatory System
QUESTION: Cardiac valves

  A: have a central core of dense fibrous connective tissue.
  B: contain both collagen and elastic fibers.
  C: are lined by endothelium on both sides.
  D: are attached to the annuli fibrosi of the cardiac skeleton.
  E: are characterized by all of the above statements.

Learning Response E: Correct. All of the above statements are true of cardiac valves.

273. SUBJECT AREA: Circulatory System
    QUESTION: Cells of the sinoatrial (SA) node

> *A:* are morphologically identical to other atrial muscle cells.
> *B:* are modified cardiac muscle cells.
> *C:* are located in the left atrium.
> *D:* are modified smooth muscle cells.
> *E:* receive electrical impulses generated by cells of the atrioventricular (AV) node.

Learning Response B: Correct. Cells of the SA node are modified cardiac muscle cells. They are smaller than atrial cells and have fewer myofibrils as well. The SA node is located in the right atrium and is the pacemaker of the heart. Thus, electrical impulses are generated in this region and then conducted by specialized cells to all the other regions of the heart.

274. SUBJECT AREA:. Circulatory System
    QUESTION: The tunica adventitia of muscular arteries is characterized by all of the following EXCEPT that it

> *A:* contains longitudinally arranged collagen and elastic fibers.
> *B:* contains large amounts of type III collagen.
> *C:* is separated from the tunica media by the external elastic lamina.
> *D:* receives nourishment from the vasa vasorum.
> *E:* may contain lymphatics and nerves.

Learning Response B: Correct. The tunica adventitia is composed of longitudinally oriented elastic and type I collagen fibers. In muscular arteries (and veins), it may also contain lymphatic channels, nerves, vasa vasorum, adipose cells, and some fibroblasts. Type III collagen is found in the tunica media. In addition, the tunica adventitia is separated from the tunica media by the external elastic lamina.

275. SUBJECT AREA: Circulatory System

QUESTION: Endothelial cells

    A: contain an abundance of microfilaments in their cytoplasm.

    B: convert bradykinin and prostaglandins to their active forms.

    C: contribute to lipogenesis.

    D: are thrombogenic.

    E: are characterized by all of the above responses.

Learning Response A: Correct. Endothelial cells are of mesenchymal origin. They line the lumenal surface of all blood vessels and exhibit a wide variety of structural alterations which allows them to serve different functions in different regions of the body. Their cytoplasm contains microfilaments. In addition, endothelial cells are metabolically active in that they can convert bradykinin and prostaglandins to *inactive* forms; they can also cleave lipoproteins into triglycerides and cholesterol. Lastly, they serve as a nonthrombogenic barrier between the subendothelial tissue and clotting factors in the blood.

276. SUBJECT AREA: Circulatory System
    QUESTION: Pericytes

    A: may function as stem cells.

    B: contain myosin, actin and tropomyosin.

    C: are a component of the tunica media of capillaries.

    D: are characterized by responses A and C above.

    E: are characterized by responses A, B and C above.

Learning Response E: Correct. Pericytes are cells of mesenchymal origin found partly surrounding endothelial cells of capillaries and venules forming the tunica media of these vessels. They may transform into other cell types. In addition, pericytes contain myosin, actin, and tropomyosin.

277. SUBJECT AREA: Circulatory System
    QUESTION: In the circulatory system,

    A: the arterial supply contains more than 70% of total

blood volume at any given time.
B: the media of medium sized veins lacks smooth
   muscle cells.
C: small and medium sized arteries (especially in the
   limbs) contain endothelium-lined valves.
D: venules may resemble capillaries in structure
   and function.
E: none of the above responses are correct.

Learning Response D: Correct. Venules contain an endothelium lined tunica
intima, a thin media of varying amounts of smooth muscle, and an adventitial
layer. The adventitia is rich in collagen fibers and is the most well developed
layer of the venule. Venules with lumenal diameters up to 50 μm are similar
to capillaries in terms of structure and biologic activity. The venous system
contains more than 70% of the total blood volume at any given time and it is
the small and medium sized veins which contain valves. Lastly, the media of
medium sized veins contains smooth muscle cells as well as reticular and
elastic fibers.

278. SUBJECT AREA: Circulatory System
       QUESTION: In the heart,

                A: the valves assist in the backward flow of blood.
                B: the endocardium, a single layer of columnar cells,
                   is analogous to the tunica adventitia of blood
                   vessels.
                C: the cardiac muscle cells, capillaries, and loose
                   connective tissue constitute the epicardium.
                D: fat is common in the myocardium.
                E: the subendocardial layer contains veins, nerves,
                   and Purkinje cells.

Learning Response E: Correct. The heart contains three layers (tunics):
endocardium, myocardium, and epicardium. The endocardium, analogous to
the tunica intima of blood vessels, is composed of a single layer of squamous
epithelial cells resting on a subendothelial layer of loose connective tissue.
Between the endocardium and myocardium is the subendocardial layer which
contains veins, nerves, and Purkinje fibers (impulse conducting cells). The
myocardium, analogous to the tunica media, is composed of cardiac

myocytes. The epicardium, analogous to the tunica adventitia, forms the visceral layer of the pericardium. Underlying the epicardium is a subepicardial layer of connective tissue which also contains veins, nerves, nerve ganglia, and adipose tissue.

---

279. SUBJECT AREA: Circulatory System
QUESTION: A person with a defect in the synthesis of type III collagen is likely to die

A: *in utero*, secondary to agenesis of the circulatory system.
B: from a defect in the tunica adventitia.
C: from an immune deficiency.
D: after a long and healthy life.
E: from a ruptured aortic aneurysm.

Learning Response E: Correct. A defect in the synthesis of type III collagen is Ehlers-Danlos syndrome. Whereas type I collagen is present in the tunica adventitia, type III collagen is present in the tunica media of blood vessels and is important in maintaining the structural integrity of the vessel. When it is absent, the strength of the media is greatly compromised and the vessel may dilate (an aneurysm), and eventually rupture. Individuals with this syndrome typically have a shortened life span secondary to this process.

---

280. SUBJECT AREA: Circulatory System
QUESTION: Identify the structure depicted in the figure below.

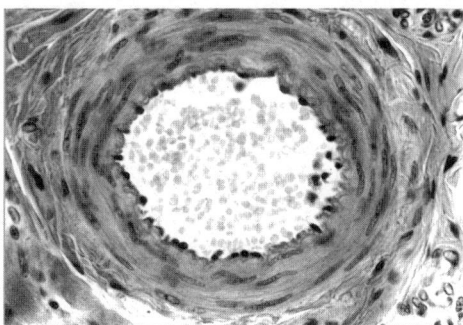

A: lymphatic vessel
B: arteriole

> *C:* elastic artery
> *D:* muscular artery
> *E:* capillary

Learning Response D: Correct. This is a small muscular or distributing artery. The endothelial cells rest on the internal elastic lamina (not clearly shown). There are three to four layers of smooth muscle cells in the tunica media which is the thickest of the three layers. The tunica adventitia blends in with the surrounding connective tissue. Lymphatic vessels and capillaries lack smooth muscle in their walls. Elastic arteries are much larger in diameter with a thick tunica media of smooth muscle and sheets of elastic fibers. Arterioles would be smaller with one or two layers of smooth muscle in the tunica media.

---

281. SUBJECT AREA: Circulatory System
QUESTION: Muscular or distributing arteries

> *A:* exhibit a well defined internal elastic lamina (IEL).
> *B:* may have skeletal muscle fibers in the tunica adventitia.
> *C:* contain 5-10 layers of smooth muscle in the tunica media.
> *D:* are lined by simple cuboidal epithelial cells.
> *E:* may contain vasa vasorum in the tunica intima.

Learning Response A: Correct. Muscular arteries contain a tunica intima which is lined (as in all vessels) by squamous endothelial cells. The intima is separated from the tunica media by a well defined IEL. The media consists of up to 40 layers of smooth muscle cells and is separated from the adventitia by the external elastic lamina. The adventitia has collagen and elastic fibers, fibroblasts, adipose tissue, lymphatic vessels, vasa vasorum and nerves and lacks skeletal muscle fibers.

---

282. SUBJECT AREA: Circulatory System
QUESTION: The endothelial cells of brain capillaries

> *A:* are fenestrated with diaphragms.
> *B:* are similar to endothelial cells found in liver capillaries.

> *C:* have numerous pinocytotic vesicles in their cytoplasm.
>
> *D:* permit the passage of most hydrophobic and some hydrophilic molecules.
>
> *E:* play a role in the formation of the blood-brain barrier.

Learning Response E: Correct. Endothelial cells of brain capillaries are continuous in that they contain no fenestrations. Other continuous capillaries include those of muscle tissue, connective tissue, and exocrine glands. While numerous pinocytotic vesicles may be found in endothelial cells of other continuous capillaries, where they transport molecules bidirectionally, they are not found in those of neural tissue. This feature helps to exclude molecules from the brain and thereby contributes to the formation of the blood-brain barrier.

283. SUBJECT AREA: Circulatory System
QUESTION: The carotid bodies

> *A:* are found near the bifurcation of the common carotid artery.
>
> *B:* are baroreceptors.
>
> *C:* are sensitive to high oxygen tension, low CO_2 concentration, and high arterial blood pH.
>
> *D:* contain abundant nerve efferent fibers.
>
> *E:* are characterized by all of the above responses.

Learning Response A: Correct. The carotid bodies are chemoreceptors found near the bifurcation of the common carotid artery. They are sensitive to low oxygen tension, high CO_2 concentration, and low arterial pH and possess afferent nerve fibers. The carotid bodies are composed of glomus cells and sheath cells.

284. SUBJECT AREA: Circulatory System
QUESTION: Glomera

> *A:* are capillaries found in the renal corpuscle.
>
> *B:* are found mainly in the face.
>
> *C:* contain no smooth muscle.

D: play an important role in regulating circulation in various organs.

E: are characterized by choices B and D above.

Learning Response D: Correct. Glomera are a complex type of arteriovenous anastomosis which are found mainly in the finger pads, fingernail beds, and ears. In addition, they are distributed throughout other organs and are thought to play a role in control of circulation and regulation of blood pressure, as well as menstruation, erection, and thermoregulation. They are innervated by both sympathetic and parasympathetic fibers. The tuft of capillaries in the renal corpuscle is known as the glomerulus.

---

285. SUBJECT AREA: Circulatory System
QUESTION: Vasa vasorum

A: are found in all peripheral blood vessels.
B: nourish cells in the tunica intima.
C: are present in large arteries only.
D: are located in the walls of large arteries and veins.
E: function to drain interstitial fluid.

Learning Response D: Correct. Vasa vasorum are small blood vessels that are located in the outer walls of large elastic arteries and large veins such as the vena cava. They provide metabolites to the tunica media and adventitia.

---

286. SUBJECT AREA: Circulatory System
QUESTION: Identify the predominant structure in the figure below.

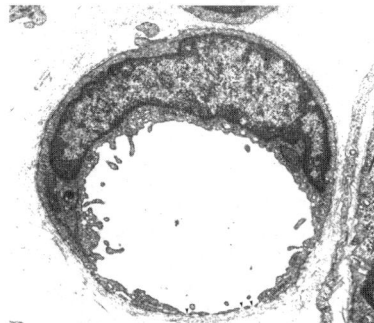

A: continuous capillary

> *B:* fenestrated capillary
> *C:* sinusoidal capillary
> *D:* lymphatic capillary
> *E:* adipose cell

Learning Response B: Correct. The thin diaphragms of the fenestrae are indicated by the arrowheads in this electron micrograph of a fenestrated capillary. Neither lymphatic capillaries nor adipose cells have these fenestrated attenuations of the cytoplasm.

---

287. SUBJECT AREA: Circulatory System
    QUESTION: Heart valvular leaflets can be considered as part of the

> *A:* endocardium.
> *B:* epicardium.
> *C:* myocardium.
> *D:* pericardium.
> *E:* subendocardial connective tissue.

Learning Response A: Correct. The valves of the heart consist of a connective tissue core and are lined on both sides by endothelial cells. Thus, they can be considered to be part of the endocardium.

---

288. SUBJECT AREA: Circulatory System
    QUESTION: The endothelial cells of continuous capillaries

> *A:* lack plasmalemmal vesicles.
> *B:* have a thin coat of smooth muscle fibers.
> *C:* are lined with macrophages.
> *D:* lack microfilaments.
> *E:* can be joined to one another by occluding junctions.

Learning Response E: Correct. The endothelial cells of continuous capillaries are held together by tight or occluding junctions which seal off the cell from the extracellular matrix. In the continuous capillaries found in the brain, the occluding junctions contribute to the blood-brain barrier which prevents noxious substances from damaging the neurons.

289. SUBJECT AREA: Circulatory System
QUESTION: Elastic arteries such as the aorta have all of the following features EXCEPT

A: a thick subendothelial layer.
B: elastic fibers in the tunica media.
C: an absence of blood vessels in the adventitia.
D: multifunctional smooth muscle cells in the media.
E: a thick tunica intima and a poorly evident internal elastic lamina.

Learning Response C: Correct. Because of the large diameter of elastic arteries, their outer wall receives nutrients from smaller blood vessels in the tunica adventitia. These blood vessels of the blood vessel are known by their Latin term vasa vasorum.

290. SUBJECT AREA: Lymphoid System
QUESTION: In the spleen,

A: the venous sinuses of the red pulp are lined by endothelial cells which are phagocytic for damaged erythrocytes.
B: the central region of the periarterial lymphatic sheaths is the domain of B lymphocytes.
C: lymphoid nodules are associated with the arterial supply.
D: the red pulp which contains venous sinuses and cellular cords is located in the medulla.
E: afferent lymphatic vessels bring lymphocytes and antigens into the organ.

Learning Response C: Correct. The spleen lacks a cortex and medulla. It is composed of white pulp consisting of lymphoid tissue embedded within red pulp which is rich in blood. The red pulp contains the cellular cords (of Billroth) and venous sinuses. Afferent lymphatic vessels are found only in lymph nodes. The phagocytic cells of the spleen are macrophages which are located mainly in the marginal zone between the red and white pulp. T lymphocytes are located primarily in the central periarterial sheaths. B lymphocytes are associated with the lymphoid nodules which are appended to the periarterial sheaths.

---

291. SUBJECT AREA: Lymphoid System
QUESTION: In the thymus,

 A: Hassall's corpuscles are restricted to the cortex.
 B: the blood-thymic barrier isolates undifferentiated lymphocytes from blood-borne antigens.
 C: medullary cords contain B lymphocytes.
 D: both afferent and efferent lymphatic vessels can be found.
 E: lobulation is best developed in adults.

Learning Response B: Correct. T lymphocytes become immunologically competent in the absence of blood-borne antigens. The connective tissue capsule of the thymus penetrates the gland and partitions it into lobules. Each lobule has a peripheral cortex and a central medulla. The cortex contains T lymphocytes, epithelial reticular cells and macrophages while the medulla houses Hassall's corpuscles, large and medium sized lymphocytes and epithelial reticular cells. Medullary cords and afferent lymphatic channels are features of lymph nodes. The thymus involutes with age, and lobulation becomes indistinct.

---

292. SUBJECT AREA: Lymphoid System
QUESTION: Which of the following statements about lymph nodes is NOT correct?

 A: Reticular fibers are one of the constituents of the stroma of the organ.
 B: Lymph nodes can be identified histologically by the presence of a subcapsular sinus.
 C: The postcapillary venules are lined with simple squamous epithelium.
 D: Blood vessels enter and leave the structure at the hilus.

E: A distinct cortex and medulla are recognizable structures.

Learning Response C: Correct. Lymphocytes enter the lymph nodes through a special type of blood vessel called postcapillary, or high endothelial, venules. These vessels are lined by tall, cuboidal endothelial cells.

---

293. SUBJECT AREA: Lymphoid System

QUESTION: All of the following structures are at least partially enclosed by a connective tissue capsule EXCEPT

A: spleen.
B: tonsil.
C: lymph node.
D: thymus.
E: solitary lymphoid nodule.

Learning Response E: Correct. Isolated or aggregated lymphoid nodules can be found in the loose connective tissue of many organs. They are surrounded by the connective tissue of the organ which is not concentrated around them such as that found in connective tissue capsules. All of the other structures have a distinct and dense capsule.

---

294. SUBJECT AREA: Lymphoid System

QUESTION: Individuals afflicted with thymic dysplasia or autosomal recessive lymphopenia (also known as DiGeorge's syndrome) have a small, vestigal thymus. All of the following would most likely be an effect of the disease EXCEPT

A: a reduction in the numbers of $CD8^+$ lymphocytes.
B: a reduction in the numbers of $CD4^+$ lymphocytes.
C: a depletion of lymphocytes from the paracortex (inner cortex) of lymph nodes.
D: a depletion of lymphocytes from the periarterial lymphatic sheaths of the spleen.
E: enlarged lymphoid nodules (follicles) in the palatine tonsil.

Learning Response E: Correct. CD8$^+$ and CD4$^+$ lymphocytes are subclasses of T lymphocytes which acquire immunocompetence in the thymus. The former are the cytotoxic T cells, and the latter are T helper cells. T lymphocytes reside in specific regions of the lymph nodes and spleen. The lymphoid nodules are mainly the domain of B lymphocytes, and a reduction in the numbers of T cells would result in impaired immune responses and a lack of enlarged tonsils.

295. SUBJECT AREA: Lymphoid System
QUESTION: In reference to humoral or antibody mediated immunity,

A: CD4$^+$ lymphocytes are usually not involved in that type of immune response.

B: the complement cascade is activated by the presence of antigen-antibody complexes at the surface of virus infected cells.

C: CD8$^+$ lymphocytes are active in the destruction of bacterial cells.

D: the activation and proliferation of lymphocytes participating in the process can occur in lymphoid nodules.

E: the secretion of interleukins by T lymphocytes activates cytotoxic T cells which destroy bacteria.

Learning Response D: Correct. B lymphocytes in lymphoid nodules are activated by interleukins produced by T helper cells (CD4$^+$ lymphocytes) resulting in the proliferation of B cells and the differentiation of some of them into plasma cells. The goal of humoral immunity is the production of antibodies, immunoglobulin molecules, which attach to bacterial cell surface antigens and mark the bacteria for destruction by macrophages or by complement enzymes.

296. SUBJECT AREA: Lymphoid System
QUESTION: The killing of virus infected somatic cells by specific cytotoxic T lymphocytes

A: results in the destruction of both the infected cell and the cytotoxic T cell.

    B: results in cytolysis and DNA fragmentation of the
       infected cell.
    C: is mediated by the activity of perforins secreted by
       the cytoxic T cell.
    D: is facilitated by the reorganization of the
       microtubule cytoskeleton of the cytotoxic T cell.
    E: is characterized by choices B, C and D above.

Learning Response E: Correct. Through the actions of cytotoxic T cells or
killer cells, virus infected somatic cells are destroyed one at a time. Only the
somatic cells are lysed and their DNA fragmented; the killer cells are not
destroyed. The microtubule cytoskeleton of the killer cells is directed to the
point of attack, and enzymes (perforins) which perforate the infected cell' s
plasma membrane are secreted.

297. SUBJECT AREA: Lymphoid System
       QUESTION: In comparing the histology of the spleen and thymus,

    A: both organs have a cortex and medulla.
    B: both organs are primary, or central, lymphoid
       organs which influence the development of
       immunocompetency of lymphocytes.
    C: afferent lymphatic vessels carry tissue fluid to the
       spleen, but not the thymus.
    D: epithelial reticular cells in the thymus are held
       together by desmosomes, and cells functionally
       similar to these are absent from the spleen.
    E: lymphoid nodules are absent from both organs.

Learning Response D: Correct. The spleen lacks a cortex and medulla and is
considered to be a secondary, or peripheral, lymphoid organ, and the thymus
is a primary, or central, lymphoid organ. Afferent lymphatic channels are only
found in lymph nodes, and lymph nodules are present in the spleen.

298. SUBJECT AREA: Lymphoid System

QUESTION: All of the following are characteristic of immunoglobulin G (IgG) EXCEPT

A: its inability to cross the placental barrier.
B: its structure of two heavy and two light weight polypeptide chains held by disulfide bonds.
C: that it is the most abundant of the serum immunoglobulins.
D: the amino terminal portions of the heavy and light chains constitute the Fab (antigen binding) fragment of the molecule.
E: it contains regions which can interact with cell surface receptors.

Learning Response A: Correct. IgG molecules are not prevented from entering the fetal circulation through the placenta. In this way they can protect the fetus and newborn infant from infection.

299. SUBJECT AREA: Lymphoid System

QUESTION: The major immunoglobulin found in tears, saliva and intestinal secretion is

A: IgM
B: IgE
C: IgG
D: IgA
E: IgD

Learning Response D: Correct. Immunoglobulin A is found in many of the secretions of the body. In addition to those listed above, it is a component of colostrum, and can also be found in nasal, bronchial, prostatic and vaginal fluids. It is found in small amounts in serum. IgG and IgM are the two major immunoglobulin components of serum, and IgM can also be located at the cell surface of B lymphocytes. IgE has an affinity for surface receptors on mast cells and basophils and functions in allergic reactions. IgD is not well characterized. It is found in low concentrations in serum and can attach to B lymphocytes along with IgM.

300. SUBJECT AREA: Lymphoid System
QUESTION: All of the following can function as antigen presenting cells EXCEPT

    A: Langerhans' cells in the epidermis.
    B: B lymphocytes.
    C: T lymphocytes.
    D: M cells (membranous epithelial cells) in the intestine.
    E: dendritic cells in lymphoid organs.

Learning Response C: Correct. There are three main classes of T lymphocytes: T helper cells (CD4$^+$ cells), T killer cells (cytotoxic T cells, CD8$^+$ cells) and T suppressor cells. Some authors consider T memory cells as a fourth class of T cells. Their diverse functions do not normally include presentation of antigen. The antigen presenting cells activate T cells as part of the immune response. The M cells are active in the immune responses of the small intestine by taking up antigens from the gut lumen and presenting them to underlying intraepithelial lymphocytes.

301. SUBJECT AREA: Lymphoid System
QUESTION: Which of the following accurately describes the flow of lymph fluid in lymph nodes?

    A: Afferent lymphatic vessel, medullary sinus, subcapsular sinus, intermediate sinus, efferent lymphatic vessel
    B: Efferent lymphatic vessel, medullary sinus, subcapsular sinus, intermediate sinus, afferent lymphatic vessel
    C: Afferent lymphatic vessel, subcapsular sinus, intermediate sinus, medullary sinus, efferent lymphatic vessel
    D: Afferent lymphatic vessel, subcapsular sinus, medullary sinus, intermediate sinus, efferent lymphatic vessel
    E: Efferent lymphatic vessel, medullary sinus, intermediate sinus, subcapsular sinus, afferent lymphatic vessel

Learning Response C: Correct. Lymph nodes are the only organs with afferent lymphatic vessels which carry lymph across the capsule and deposit it in the subcapsular sinus. From there lymph flows in the intermediate sinuses that run along the connective tissue trabeculae in the interior of the lymph node. The intermediate sinuses communicate with the medullary sinuses and drain into the efferent lymphatic vessels which transport lymph away from the node.

---

302. SUBJECT AREA: Lymphoid System

QUESTION: All of the following are functions of the spleen EXCEPT

> *A:* the removal of damaged or effete erythrocytes.
> *B:* the formation of leukocytes and erythrocytes.
> *C:* the breakdown of hemoglobin into its components.
> *D:* the immune response to antigens.
> *E:* phagocytosis of bacteria as well as inert material in the blood.

Learning Response B: Correct. In the adult, the spleen is not a blood forming organ, but acts as a filter of blood by removing damaged or worn out red blood cells, as well as bacteria and inert particles that may be found in the blood stream. In the destruction of erythrocytes, macrophages in the spleen break down hemoglobin into the iron-containing heme component and the globin protein. Globin is hydrolyzed into amino acids which are reused in protein synthesis. Iron is released from heme and transported in the blood stream, and heme is converted into bilirubin which is carried to the liver and excreted in bile.

---

303. SUBJECT AREA: Lymphoid System

QUESTION: The palatine tonsils

> *A:* are covered by stratified squamous epithelium.
> *B:* contain epithelial invaginations or crypts.
> *C:* are separated from subjacent structures by a connective tissue capsule.
> *D:* contain numerous lymphoid nodules underlying the epithelial tisssue.

*

E: can be characterized by all of the above features.

Learning Response E: Correct. The palatine tonsils located in the lateral walls of the oropharynx are important in the protection of the oral cavity from bacterial infections and have all of the above features.

304. SUBJECT AREA: Lymphoid System

QUESTION: The epithelial reticular cells of the thymus

A: are located mainly in the connective tissue capsule.

B: consist of widely separated individual cells.

C: contain bundles of cytoskeletal filaments composed primarily of actin.

D: are not considered to be part of the blood-thymus barrier.

E: are stellate cells held together by desmosomes forming a cellular network.

Learning Response E: Correct. As part of the blood-thymus barrier, the epithelial reticular cells in the thymic cortex constitute a cellular network that isolates developing T cells from blood-borne antigens. The cells have adherent junctions formed by desmosomes and have bundles of cytokeratin intermediate filaments.

305. SUBJECT AREA: Lymphoid System

QUESTION: Cellular immunity, also called cell mediated immunity, has all of the following characteristics EXCEPT

A: destruction of virus infected somatic cells.

B: formation of molecules that circulate in the blood stream to inactivate or destroy bacteria.

C: destruction of tumor cells.

D: the ability to reject tissue grafts.

E: production of memory T cells.

Learning Response B: Correct. Cellular immunity does not involve the production of antibody molecules or immunoglobulins which circulate in the fluids of the body to render harmless any foreign invader. This is the realm of humoral immunity in which activated B cells differentiate into plasma cells which secrete the immunoglobulins.

---

306. SUBJECT AREA: Lymphoid System
QUESTION: Antigens are foreign substances which elicit an immune response and can be

  A: protein molecules.
  B: foreign cells.
  C: cell surface polysaccharides.
  D: nucleoproteins.
  E: all of the above possibilities.

Learning Response E: Correct. Antigens can be anything which is foreign to the host and capable of initiating an immune response. All of the above have features called antigenic determinants which can be recognized as foreign to the body.

---

307. SUBJECT AREA: Lymphoid System
QUESTION: In allergic reactions, mast cells or basophils sensitized to pollen have which of the following immunoglobulins at their surface?

  A: IgA
  B: IgD
  C: IgE
  D: IgG
  E: IgM

Learning Response C: Correct. In the first encounter with antigenic pollen, plasma cells derived from activated B lymphocytes produce IgE which quickly disappears from circulation as it attaches itself to receptors at the plasma membrane of basophils and mast cells. Subsequent attacks result in the rapid degranulation of these cells releasing a number of vasoactive substances including histamine and heparin.

308. SUBJECT AREA: Lymphoid System
QUESTION: Hassall's corpuscles

A: are located in the lamina propria of the ileum as a component of Peyer's patches.
B: consist of degenerating, flattened epithelial reticular cells.
C: are arterioles located in the thymic medulla.
D: are characteristic of the white pulp of the spleen.
E: consist of dendritic cells in the medulla of lymph nodes.

Learning Response B: Correct. Hassall's corpuscles are structures characteristic of the thymic medulla and consist of concentrically arranged, degenerating epithelial reticular cells that contain keratohyalin granules.

309. SUBJECT AREA: Lymphoid System
QUESTION: The major difference between primary and secondary lymphoid nodules is that the

A: latter are located in the secondary lymphoid organs (spleen, lymph nodes, etc.) while the former are confined to the primary lymphoid organs (thymus or bone marrow).
B: latter contain a germinal center which is a clear zone containing immunoblast cells.
C: latter contain lymphocytes and antigen presenting cells while the former do not possess these cells.
D: former represent exposure to antigen and the latter have not been antigenically stimulated.
E: latter are located in the medulla of lymph nodes while the former are found in the cortex.

Learning Response B: Correct. Primary lymphoid nodules are spherical accumulations of lymphocytes with no clear central regions. These structures appear in lymph nodes which have not been exposed to antigen. Secondary nodules have a clear, central zone in which are located immunoblast cells resulting from antigenic stimulation. The primary lymphoid organs, thymus

and bone marrow, lack nodules of lymphocytes. In the lymph nodes, the
nodules are restricted to the cortex.

---

310. SUBJECT AREA: Lymphoid System
QUESTION: The periarterial lymphatic sheaths of the spleen

A: are associated with the trabecular arteries.
B: constitute the adventitia of the venous sinuses.
C: are components of the splenic (Billroth's) cords.
D: function in the removal of damaged erythrocytes.
E: are collections of lymphocytes in the adventitia of
the central arteries.

Learning Response E: Correct. As part of the white pulp of the spleen, the
periarterial lymphatic sheaths consist of lymphocytes which are located in the
tunica adventitia of the central arteries as they emerge from the trabeculae.
Often lymphoid nodules are associated with these vessels such that the artery
occupies an eccentric location, and yet retains its name as the central artery.
The cords and venous sinuses constitute the red pulp of the spleen.

---

311. SUBJECT AREA: Lymphoid System
QUESTION: Which of the following types of tissue or organ
transplants are least likely to be rejected by the
immune cells of the host?

A: autografts and homografts
B: homografts and heterografts
C: isografts and autografts
D: isografts and homografts
E: autografts and heterografts

Learning Response C: Correct. When the transplanted material is taken from
different sites of the host, the transplant is called an autograft. When taken
from an identical twin, the transplant is an isograft. These two types of
transplants are the least likely to be rejected by the host. Homografts are
taken from an individual of the same species as the host, and heterografts are
transplanted from a different species. These last two have cells with surface
receptors that do not entirely match those of the host, and, as a result, the

host's immune system can reject the transplants.

---

312. SUBJECT AREA: Lymphoid System
        QUESTION: Identify the organ shown in the figure below.

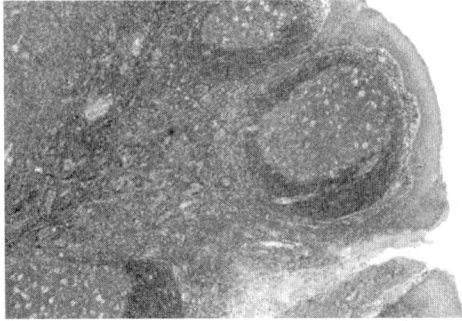

A: lymph node
B: thymus
C: spleen
D: palatine tonsil
E: pharyngeal tonsil

Learning Response D: Correct. The palatine tonsils are covered by stratified squamous epithelium under which lie several lymphoid nodules. The pharyngeal tonsil typically has pseudostratified ciliated epithelium at its surface and lacks crypts. The lymph node, thymus and spleen all have a dense connective tissue capsule at their surface.

---

313. SUBJECT AREA: Lymphoid System
        QUESTION: Identify the organ shown in the figure below.

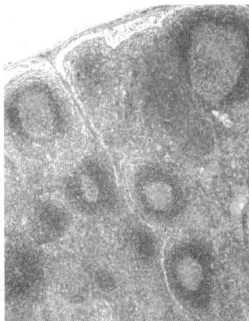

> *A:* lymph node
> *B:* spleen
> *C:* thymus
> *D:* bone marrow
> *E:* lingual tonsil

Learning Response A: Correct. Just below the connective tissue capsule is the subcapsular or marginal sinus, a key histological feature in the identification of lymph nodes. None of the other organs has such a sinus. The cortex of the lymph node contains numerous lymphoid nodules, and the medulla is located at the lower portion of the micrograph.

---

314. SUBJECT AREA: Lymphoid System

QUESTION: In the figure below, identify the lightly stained cells in this section through the thymus.

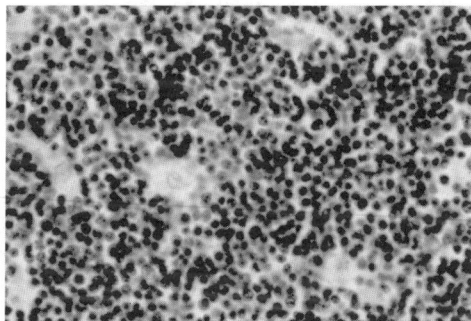

> *A:* lymphocytes
> *B:* pericytes
> *C:* epithelial reticular cells
> *D:* dendritic cells
> *E:* endothelial cellc

Learning Response C: Correct. Epithelial reticular cells are components of the blood-thymus barrier which allows the development of T lymphocytes in the absence of antigens. The endothelial cells of capillaries and the thick basement membrane between the endothelial cells and the epithelial reticular cells are also part of the structure.

315. SUBJECT AREA: Integumentary System
QUESTION: Touch receptors in the papillary layer of the dermis are

A: Merkel's cells.
B: Pacinian corpuscles.
C: free nerve endings.
D: Meissner's corpuscles.
E: Langerhans' cells.

Learning Response D: Correct. Merkel's cells, free nerve endings and Langerhans' cells are located in the epidermis. Pacinian corpuscles are usually found in the deeper layers of the dermis. All except Langerhans' cells, which are antigen presenting cells, are sensory endings.

316. SUBJECT AREA: Integumentary System
QUESTION: The secretory portions of eccrine sweat glands are usually located

A: in the stratum corneum.
B: in the stratum basale.
C: in the papillary layer of the dermis.
D: in the dermis adjacent to hair follicles.
E: deep in the dermis near the subcutaneous tissue.

Learning Response E: Correct. The secretory portions of eccrine sweat glands are found deep in the dermis. The ducts from these glands course through all layers of the dermis and epidermis.

317. SUBJECT AREA Integumentary System
QUESTION: The epidermis

A: derives its nourishment from capillaries in the stratum spinosum.
B: serves as location sites for Pacinian corpuscles.
C: is the innermost layer of the skin.

D: rests on an underlying basal lamina.
E: is typically not keratinized.

Learning Response D: Correct. The epidermis consists of keratinized stratified squamous epithelium and lacks capillaries. As an epithelium, the epidermis rests on a basal lamina and is supported by the underlying connective tissue of the dermis.

318. SUBJECT AREA: Integumentary System
QUESTION: Appendages to skin (hair or nails)

A: are keratinized.
B: are found in both thin and thick skin.
C: contain non-nucleated cells.
D: are derived from ectoderm.
E: exhibit all of the above features.

Learning Response E: Correct. Both hair and nails are keratinized with non-nucleated cells at the periphery. Hair is found on thin skin; nails on thick skin, and both are derived from ectodermal tissue.

319. SUBJECT AREA: Integumentary System
QUESTION: Melanocytes

A: are increased in individuals with dark skin.
B: are of mesodermal origin.
C: contain cytoplasmic extensions which deliver melanin to the stratum corneum and stratum lucidum.
D: contain vesicles which demonstrate tyrosinase activity.
E: are attached to surrounding keratinocytes by desmosomes.

Learning Response D: Correct. Tyrosinase activity is required in the developing melanin granule for the initial conversion of tyrosine to dopa. A multi-step process then converts dopa to melanin in the mature melanin granule. The number of melanocytes per unit area is the same in all humans; the number of melanin granules deposited in the keratinocytes determines degree of pigmentation. Melanocytes are of neural crest origin and deliver mature melanin granules to cells in the stratum basale and stratum spinosum. Melanocytes are not attached to keratinocytes but are bonded to the basal lamina via hemidesmosomes.

320. SUBJECT AREA: Integumentary System
QUESTION: The layers of keratinocytes in thick skin, from superficial to deep, are

> *A:* corneum, lucidum, spinosum, granulosum, basale.
> *B:* corneum, granulosum, lucidum, basale, spinosum.
> *C:* lucidum, corneum, spinosum, granulosum, basale.
> *D:* corneum, spinosum, basale, lucidum, granulosum.
> *E:* corneum, lucidum, granulosum, spinosum, basale.

Learning Response E: Correct. Both thick and thin skin have the same layers, although the stratum lucidum is more prominent in thick skin. Thick skin is generally hairless and found on the palms and soles while thin skin can have hair follicles and is found on the rest of the body. The terms thick and thin refer only to the thickness of the epidermal layer. Thus, skin on the back is classified as thin even though dermal and epidermal thickness combined may be 4 mm (the epidermal component is only 75–150 μm).

321. SUBJECT AREA: Integumentary System
QUESTION: Thin skin

> *A:* is characterized by a prominent stratum lucidum.
> *B:* is characterized by an avascular epidermis.
> *C:* contains no hair follicles.
> *D:* is found on the palms and soles.
> *E:* has no underlying dermis.

Learning Response B: Correct. Both thick and thin skin contain no blood vessels. The epidermis receives its nutrients from the underlying vascular dermis. Thin skin has a less prominent stratum lucidum than thick skin, contains hair follicles, and is found everywhere on the body except the palms and soles.

---

322. SUBJECT AREA: Integumentary System
QUESTION: Langerhans' cells

> *A:* are the dominant epidermal cell type.
> *B:* have long cytoplasmic processes terminating in the stratum basale and stratum spinosum.
> *C:* play a role in immune responses of the integumentary system.
> *D:* may serve as mechanoreceptors.
> *E:* are of neural crest origin.

Learning Response C: Correct. Langerhans' cells function in antigen presentation to T lymphocytes and are, therefore, an important component of the skin's immunologic defenses. They comprise only 2–8% of the epidermis, while the keratinocytes are the dominant epidermal cell type. Langerhans' cells are bone marrow derivatives. Melanocytes are of neural crest origin and have long cytoplasmic processes terminating in the strata basale and spinosum. Merkel's cells are thought to function as mechanoreceptors.

---

323. SUBJECT AREA: Integumentary System
QUESTION: The reticular layer of the dermis

> *A:* is classified as dense irregular connective tissue.
> *B:* is classified as loose connective tissue.
> *C:* contains a rich capillary network with thermoregulatory functions.
> *D:* lacks fibroblasts.
> *E:* forms projections which help anchor the dermis to the epidermis.

Learning Response A: Correct. The reticular layer of the dermis is composed of dense irregular connective tissue, mostly type I collagen. The rest of the responses describe the more superficial papillary layer of the dermis.

324. SUBJECT AREA: Integumentary System
QUESTION: Hair follicles

A: arise from invaginations of the epidermis.
B: derive nutrients from basally located dermal papillae.
C: rest on an underlying basal lamina.
D: are surrounded by a connective tissue sheath to which arrector pili muscles may attach.
E: have all of the above features.

Learning Response E: Correct. All of the above responses are true of hair follicles.

325. SUBJECT AREA: Integumentary System
QUESTION: The skin

A: may give rise to tumors of ectodermal origin.
B: may give rise to tumors of keratinocyte origin.
C: may give rise to tumors of neural crest origin.
D: may blister if cell to cell adhesions between keratinocytes are disrupted.
E: may be characterized by all of the above.

Learning Response E: Correct. Tumors in the skin may arise from keratinocytes, which are of ectodermal origin. These tumors include basal cell carcinoma and squamous cell carcinoma. Melanocytes are of neural crest origin and may give rise to malignant melanoma. Bullous (blistering) diseases of the skin may arise from disorders in the dermal-epidermal junction (bullous pemphigoid) or from disorders in cell to cell adhesions within the epidermis (pemphigus vulgaris).

326. SUBJECT AREA: Integumentary System
QUESTION: In regard to nails,

A: the nail bed contains all five cell layers of epidermis.

B: nail plate epithelium is derived from the nail matrix.

C: cells in the nail plate are equivalent to cells of the stratum basale.

D: the fingernail is formed from the underlying nail bed.

E: all of the above are true.

Learning Response B: Correct. The nail plate epithelium is derived from the nail matrix at the proximal end of the nail, not from a maturation of underlying cells of the nail bed. The fold of skin overlying the nail root does contain all normal layers of the epidermis but the cells of the nail plate correspond to the keratinized cells of the stratum corneum. The nail bed only contains cells of the stratum basale and stratum spinosum.

327. SUBJECT AREA: Integumentary System
QUESTION: All of the following statements are true EXCEPT

A: hair follicles contain nerve endings for the sense of touch.

B: dermal papillae contain a rich vascular supply.

C: eccrine sweat gland ducts open into the upper portion of the hair follicle.

D: apocrine sweat glands are present in the groin, axilla, and areola.

E: the secretory portion of eccrine sweat glands is found in the dermis and is surrounded by myoepithelial cells.

Learning Response C: Correct. Sebaceous glands secrete sebum into the upper portion of the hair follicle; in regions such as the lips, glans clitoris, and glans penis, the secretion is directly onto the skin surface. While apocrine sweat glands also open into hair follicles, eccrine sweat glands have ducts which open only on the skin surface.

328. SUBJECT AREA: Integumentary System
QUESTION: Sebaceous glands

A: are found primarily in thick skin.

B: are holocrine glands.

C: secrete fluid composed primarily of protein and water.

D: are located in the stratum basale.

E: have all of the above features.

Learning Response B: Correct. Sebaceous glands are examples of holocrine glands because their secretory product, sebum, contains dead glandular cells. The glands are found in the dermis. However, they are not found in the palms and soles because those areas are covered by (hairless) thick skin. Sebum is composed primarily of lipid.

329. SUBJECT AREA: Integumentary System
QUESTION: Renewal of the epidermis

A: takes 15–30 days.

B: is due to proliferation in the stratum lucidum and stratum corneum.

C: is dependent upon nutrients received from capillaries in the reticular layer of the dermis.

D: results in an outermost layer, the stratum corneum, which is composed of flattened, nucleated, keratinized cells.

E: is characterized by all of the above choices.

Learning Response A: Correct. Constant renewal of the epidermis is due to mitotic activity in the stratum basale and the lower portion of the stratum spinosum. (The area in which all mitoses occur is termed the malpighian layer.) The process results in a stratum corneum composed of flattened, keratinized, non-nucleated cells. Capillaries in the dermal papillae provide the blood supply to the epidermis.

330. SUBJECT AREA: Integumentary System
QUESTION: Keratohyalin granules are characteristic of cells in the

A: stratum corneum.
B: stratum spinosum.
C: stratum lucidum.
D: stratum basale.
E: stratum granulosum.

Learning Response E: Correct. The stratum granulosum contains keratohyalin granules, which are not membrane-bound and contain large amounts of basophilic phosphate groups. The cells of this layer also have lamellar granules which are lipid-rich. The contents of the lamellar granules when deposited into the extracellular space function to seal those areas between cells thus providing a barrier to foreign particle movements in the skin. The stratum granulosum itself is only 3–5 cells thick and composed of flattened polygonal cells with centrally placed nuclei.

331. SUBJECT AREA: Integumentary System
QUESTION: Lamellar granules are characteristic of cells in the

A: stratum corneum.
B: stratum spinosum.
C: stratum lucidum.
D: stratum basale.
E: stratum granulosum.

Learning Response E: Correct. The cells of the stratum granulosum contain lamellar granules which have lipid material. When the contents of the granules are secreted into the intercellular spaces of the stratum granulosum, they seal off that area and, as a result, play an integral part in allowing the skin to act as barrier to environmental pathogens and other agents. The cells in this layer also contain keratohyalin granules.

332. SUBJECT AREA: Integumentary System
QUESTION: Identify the structure shown in the figure below.

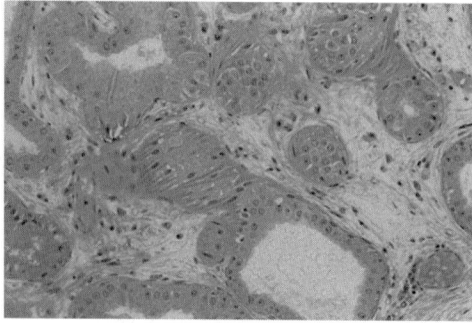

A: sebaceous gland
B: apocrine sweat gland
C: mucus secreting gland
D: eccrine sweat gland
E: eccrine sweat duct

Learning Response B: Correct. Apocrine sweat glands are located in the axilla, the areolae and the anus. They are generally larger in diameter than eccrine sweat glands. Sebaceous glands are associated with hair follicles and contain lipid. Some of the myoepithelial cells of the apocrine are visible in this micrograph.

333. SUBJECT AREA: Integumentary System
QUESTION: In the figure below, destruction of cell to cell adhesions would result in

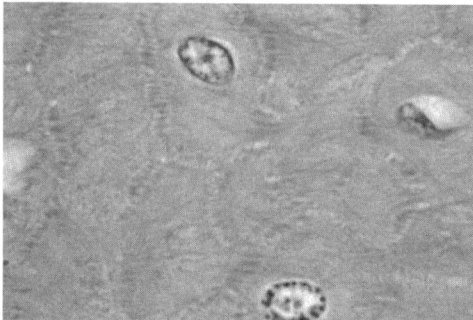

A: an immune deficiency.
B: vitiligo.

C: blistering.
D: albinism.
E: psoriasis.

Learning Response C: Correct. The micrograph depicts a section of the stratum spinosum and shows the characteristic cytoplasmic extensions, intercellular bridges, and cytoplasmic tonofibrils. If these intercellular connections, which correspond to spot desmosomes in electron micrographs, are disrupted (e.g., by friction or by autoantibodies), blisters will result. Albinism results from an inability of melanocytes to synthesize melanin, whereas vitiligo is caused by the loss of melanocytes. Psoriasis is a common dermatologic condition characterized by a rapid turnover of keratinocytes.

334. SUBJECT AREA: Integumentary System
QUESTION: In the figure below, identify the cytoskeletal structures indicated by the arrows.

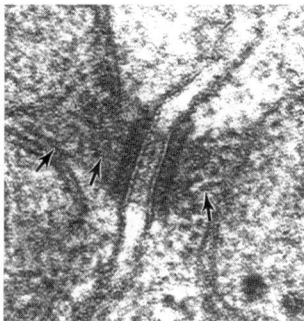

A: tonofilaments
B: mictrotubules
C: type IV collagen
D: microfilaments
E: myosin filaments

Learning Response A: Correct. Desmosomes are numerous in the lateral and upper surfaces of cells of the stratum basale and function in attachment to surrounding keratinocytes. These structures consist of thickened plasma membranes of each cell into which are inserted cytokeratin intermediate filaments which are also known as tonofilaments. Microfilaments are not components of desmosomes. Microtubules provide the basis for several cytoplasmic components, including centrioles, basal bodies, cilia, and flagella. Type IV collagen is present in the basal lamina and does not contribute to the formation of desmosomes.

---

335. SUBJECT AREA: Integumentary System
QUESTION: All of the following are components of the epidermis EXCEPT

A: hair follicles.
B: Meissner's corpuscles.
C: nails.
D: keratin.
E: sebaceous glands.

Learning Response B: Correct. Meissner's corpuscles are found in the dermis of the skin of the palms, soles, nipples, and lips. They respond to tactile stimuli. Other sensory structures in the dermis include Pacinian corpuscles and Ruffini's endings. All the other choices are components of the epidermis. Hair follicles, which arise from epidermal invaginations, are associated with unmyelinated fibers that sense touch.

---

336. SUBJECT AREA: Integumentary System
QUESTION: Structures which help to anchor the epidermis to the basal lamina include

A: microtubules.
B: desmosomes.
C: Langerhans' cells.
D: hemidesmosomes.
E: the lamina reticularis.

Learning Response D: Correct. Hemidesmosomes in the epidermis are specifically found in the basal plasmalemma of cells of the stratum basale and serve to bind these cells to the underlying basal lamina. Desmosomes are found throughout the epidermis and form cell to cell adhesions. Langerhans' cells are the antigen presenting cells of the epidermis and play no role in cell to cell adhesions. The lamina reticularis is a net of reticular fibers which underlies the basal lamina. The basal lamina and lamina reticularis are collectively known as the basement membrane.

337. SUBJECT AREA: Integumentary System
QUESTION: Arrector pili muscles are composed of

> *A:* skeletal muscle.
> *B:* cardiac muscle.
> *C:* smooth muscle.
> *D:* both skeletal and smooth muscle.
> *E:* both cardiac and skeletal muscle.

Learning Response C: Correct. Arrector pili muscles are composed only of smooth muscle fibers. They link the connective tissue sheath that surrounds the hair follicle to the papillary layer of the dermis.

338. SUBJECT AREA: Integumentary System
QUESTION: Eccrine sweat glands

> *A:* have ducts which open at the skin surface.
> *B:* are located in the stratum basale.
> *C:* are present in the axillary, areolar and anal regions.
> *D:* have ducts which open into hair follicles.
> *E:* are characterized by all of the above features.

Learning Response A: Correct. Eccrine sweat glands are simple, coiled tubular glands whose secretory portions are located in the dermis. Their ducts open at the skin surface. Eccrine sweat glands secrete a nonviscous fluid which is composed primarily of water, sodium chloride, urea, ammonia and uric acid. Apocrine sweat glands are modified sweat glands present in the axillary, areolar, and anal regions. They are much larger than eccrine sweat glands and secrete a viscous fluid.

339. SUBJECT AREA: Integumentary System

QUESTION: The following can serve to distinguish thick skin from thin skin EXCEPT

    A: hair follicles are only in thin skin.

    B: the presence of a more apparent stratum lucidum in thick skin.

    C: the absence of the stratum spinosum in thick skin.

    D: the thickened stratum corneum of thick skin.

    E: the presence of arrector pili muscles only in thin skin.

Learning Response C: Correct. All five layers of the epidermis are present in both thick and thin skin. However, the more prominent stratum lucidum of thick skin (choice B) is a valuable differential clue, as are choices A, D, and E.

340. SUBJECT AREA: Endocrine System

QUESTION: If the inhibitory feedback mechanism is disrupted, as in ovariectomy, the gonadotrophic cells in the pituitary will

    A: stop secreting gonadotropin releasing hormone (GnRH).

    B: continue to synthesize luteinizing hormone (LH).

    C: atrophy.

    D: stop secreting prolactin.

    E: increase the secretion of oxytocin.

Learning Response B: Correct. Gonadotrophic cell secretion is inhibited by increasing levels of circulating estrogen and progesterone from the ovary; ovariectomy removes this inhibitory feedback mechanism and the cells continue to release LH and FSH.

341. SUBJECT AREA: Endocrine System

QUESTION: An increase in dopaminergic secretion from the hypothalamic arcuate nucleus will result in

A: an increase in prolactin releasing hormone.
B: a decrease in prolactin inhibiting factor.
C: a decrease in pituitary prolactin secretion.
D: an increase in pituitary prolactin secretion.
E: an increase in the feedback inhibition of dopamine by prolactin.

Learning Response C: Correct. Arcuate nucleus dopamine is the definitive prolactin inhibitory factor; without the neurotransmitter dopamine, prolactin is tonically released from pituitary lactotrophs. Other neurohormones–neurotransmitters (such as VIP, oxytocin, other catecholamines) only modulate the prolactin inhibitory effect of dopaminE: In addition, neither a true prolactin inhibitory factor (PIF) neuropeptide nor a prolactin releasing factor has been biochemically characterized or anatomically localized yet.

342. SUBJECT AREA: Endocrine System

QUESTION: The hormonal content of anterior pituitary cells can be specifically identified by all of the following EXCEPT

A: acidophilic or basophilic staining characteristics.
B: immunocytochemistry.
C: granular size.
D: electron opacity of granular content.
E: fibrous bodies.

Learning Response A: Correct. Chromatophilia cannot specifically identify hormone content and the term is no longer relevant to cytologic or pathologic diagnosis. Fibrous bodies, found only in somatotrophic cells, are composed of intermediate filaments and organelle debris; they are indicative of a benign somatotropic adenoma resulting in acromegaly.

343. SUBJECT AREA: Endocrine System
QUESTION: The precursor neurohormone, proopiomelanocortin (POMC), is

A: proteolytically converted to neurophysin and vasopressin.
B: proteolytically converted to β-lipotropin and corticotropin releasing hormone (CRH).
C: found exclusively in the pars nervosa.
D: produced by somatotrophic cells.
E: found in the fetal and neonatal pituitary only.

Learning Response B: Correct. Differential processing of a preprohormone depends on availability of tissue-specific enzymes. Corticotrophs in the pars distalis and intermediate lobe of the pituitary enzymatically process the preprohormone POMC into ACTH, beta-lipotropin, beta-endorphin or alpha-MSH. Neurophysin is a binding protein for vasopressin and oxytocin.

344. SUBJECT AREA: Endocrine System
QUESTION: A major difference between neurotransmitter-containing neurons and neurohormone-containing neurons is that

A: neurotransmitter neurons always synapse with other neurons.
B: neuroendocrine neurons synapse only on pituitary cells.
C: the relatively long half-life of neurohormones allows them to affect distant targets.
D: neurotransmitters are usually released into the blood stream to affect target nuclei.
E: neuropeptide neurons do not have a paracrine effect on nearby neurons.

Learning Response C: Correct. Neurons containing neurotransmitters can and do synapse on neuropeptide-containing neurons, as well as blood vessels, muscle, etc. Neuropeptide neurons can have a paracrine effect on nearby neurons throughout the brain, as well as direct synaptic transmission.

---

345. SUBJECT AREA: Endocrine System

QUESTION: In the pars nervosa,

A: oxytocinergic neurons synapse on chromophobes.

B: antidiuretic hormone (ADH, vasopressin) is released from axon terminals of neurons originating in both the supraoptic (SON) and paraventricular (PVN) nuclei.

C: Herring bodies containing proopiomelanocortin (POMC) are located there.

D: pituicytes store and release vasopressin.

E: the internal carotid branches into portal capillaries.

Learning Response B: Correct. Vasopressinergic neurons synthesizing ADH and projecting axons to the posterior pituitary originate in both the SON and PVN. Pituicytes are glial cells and do not synthesize vasopressin. The inferior hypophyseal artery supplies blood to the neurohypophysis; portal capillaries are located in the adenohypophysis.

---

346. SUBJECT AREA: Endocrine System

QUESTION: In a congenital defect involving the neural tube, should the infant survive, the component(s) of the hypophysis affected would be

A: both pars nervosa and pars distalis.

B: the infundibulum and pars nervosa.

C: the intermediate lobe and the anterior lobe.

D: the adenohypophysis only.

E: the intermediate lobe only.

Learning Response B: Correct. The other components are derived from the oral ectoderm of Rathke's pouch. The infundibulum and pars nervosa develop from the floor of the diencephalon, not the neural tube.

---

347. SUBJECT AREA: Endocrine System

QUESTION: Vasopressin (antidiuretic hormone, ADH)

A: is secreted from the neurohypophysis when the osmotic pressure of blood decreases.

B: decreases the permeability of renal collecting tubules to water.

C: regulates osmotic balance.

D: is primarily responsible for blood pressure homeostasis.

E: is involved in uterine contraction during childbirth.

Learning Response C: Correct. ADH increases the uptake of water from the collecting ducts, thereby concentrating the urine and preventing water loss (diuresis); it is secreted in response to an increase in osmotic pressure. Oxytocin secretions from the neurohypophysis function in stimulating uterine contractions during parturition.

348. SUBJECT AREA: Endocrine System

QUESTION: The median eminence is an important site because it is

A: an anatomical landmark for the supraoptic nucleus.

B: the remnant of Rathke's pouch.

C: the site where neuroendocrine neurons synapse on portal capillaries.

D: the connection between the hypothalamic nuclei and the pars nervosa.

E: a major constituent of the blood-brain barrier.

Learning Response C: Correct. The median eminence is the site where hypothalamic releasing or inhibiting factors are secreted into the portal vessels to act on cells in the adenohypophysis (pars distalis). It is one of the few sites in the brain where the blood-brain barrier is "leaky," allowing compounds in systemic circulation access to the axon terminals that synapse there.

349. SUBJECT AREA: Endocrine System

QUESTION: The excessive water loss seen with diabetes insipidus is the result of the inactivity or loss of

A: vasopressinergic neurons in the hypothalamus.

    B: lactotrophic cells in the pars nervosa.

    C: vasopressin secretion from the pars distalis.

    D: glucoregulatory responses in the adrenal cortex in response to ACTH from the anterior pituitary.

    E: insulin deficient receptors on somatotrophic cells.

Learning Response A: Correct. Antidiuretic hormone or ADH, another name for vasopressin, is secreted from the pars nervosa of the pituitary, but the cell bodies are located in the hypothalamus.

350. SUBJECT AREA: Endocrine System

    QUESTION: The hypophyseal portal system is a capillary bed

    A: that provides vascular supply and drainage inside the hypothalamus.

    B: on which neurohormone-containing axons synapse inside the hypothalamus.

    C: that connects the median eminence with the pituitary.

    D: that conducts oxytocin and vasopressin to the neurohypophysis.

    E: with bidirectional flow, so that pituitary hormones can affect hypothalamic neurons.

Learning Response C: Correct. Portal synaptic connections are not located within the hypothalamus, but at its ventral surface; flow is unidirectional.

351. SUBJECT AREA: Endocrine System

    QUESTION: Elevated blood levels of a hormone from a target organ can reduce or inhibit the continued effect of a specific pituitary hormone via all of the following mechanisms EXCEPT direct

    A: inhibition of specific hypothalamic releasing factors.

    B: inhibition of specific pituitary releasing factors.

    C: stimulation of specific hypothalamic inhibiting factors.

D: inhibition of the specific pituitary hormone.

E: stimulation of neurons with inhibitory input to the pituitary cell.

Learning Response B: Correct. There are no "pituitary" releasing factors, only hypothalamic releasing factors.

---

352. SUBJECT AREA: Endocrine System

QUESTION: In regard to hypothalamic effects on the pituitary,

A: all hypothalamic factors have stimulatory effects on the pituitary.

B: hypothalamic control of the pituitary is exclusively through the portal capillary system.

C: the only hypothalamic nuclei involved are the supraoptic nucleus (SON) and paraventricular nucleus (PVN).

D: hypothalamic neurons can synapse directly on pituitary cells.

E: feedback from the pituitary hormones can inhibit further hypothalamic effects.

Learning Response E: Correct. Hypothalamic control of the pituitary occurs via the axons from multiple different nuclei projecting to either 1) the portal capillaries for secretion of both inhibitory and releasing factors, or 2) the neurohypophysis where secretory products (ADH, oxytocin, neurophysin) are stored in dilations of the terminals called Herring bodies for release into capillaries. Pituitary hormone feedback can inhibit hypothalamic secretion (ultra-short inhibitory feedback loop).

---

353. SUBJECT AREA: Endocrine System

QUESTION: Hypophysectomy results in

A: loss of direct adrenal stimulation by corticotropin releasing hormone (CRH).

B: adrenal cortical atrophy.

C: adrenal cortical hypertrophy.

D: adrenal medullary hypertrophy.

E: adrenal medullary atrophy.

Learning Response B: Correct. Hypophysectomy of the pituitary removes ACTH stimulation of adrenocortical cells, resulting in atrophy. The surgery would not remove hypothalamic CRH, which acts on pituitary corticotrophs, not adrenocortical cells. Neither CRH nor ACTH affects adrenomedullary cells.

---

354. SUBJECT AREA: Endocrine System
QUESTION: In regard to antidiuretic hormone,

A: its secretion is stimulated by a high intake of water.
B: it decreases the permeability of the kidney tubules to water.
C: it affects the renal proximal convoluted tubules.
D: it causes the formation of hypotonic urine.
E: it is essential in water conservation after diarrhea or excessive sweating.

Learning Response E: Correct. All other choices involve a loss of water from the body; ADH functions to conserve water.

---

355. SUBJECT AREA: Endocrine System
QUESTION: All of the following are true about oxytocin EXCEPT

A: it is present in males.
B: it is stored in Herring bodies.
C: its release can be stimulated by the neurohormonal milk-ejection reflex.
D: a reduction in secretion results in diabetes mellitus.
E: neurons producing it are found in both the supraoptic and paraventricular nuclei of the hypothalamus.

Learning Response D: Correct. Diabetes mellitus is a disorder of glucose regulation. Diabetes insipidus, due to the loss of vasopressinergic neurons, is an inability to concentrate urine. Oxytocin is present in males, but its function, like that of prolactin, is undetermined.

356. SUBJECT AREA: Endocrine System
QUESTION: In humans, prolactin functions to

A: maintain the corpus luteum.
B: initiate proliferation of unprimed lactiferous ducts.
C: maintain milk secretion.
D: initiate mammary growth at puberty.
E: maintain prostatic submucosal glands.

Learning Response C: Correct. Prolactin has no effect on human corpus luteum. Estrogen and progesterone are responsible for growth of the mammary gland; prolactin has little effect on an unprimed gland. The action of prolactin in males has not been determined yet.

357. SUBJECT AREA: Endocrine System
QUESTION: The hypothalamo-hypophyseal neuronal tract

A: connects the adenohypophysis with the neurohypophysis.
B: connects Rathke's pouch with the hypothalamus.
C: is a passageway for releasing factors to the adenohypophysis.
D: connects the adenohypophysis with the hypothalamus.
E: is a passageway for oxytocin and vasopressin (antidiuretic hormone, ADH) to the neurohypophysis.

Learning Response E: Correct. Oxytocin and vasopressin are synthesized by cells in the supraoptic and paraventricular nuclei of the hypothalamus, packaged into small secretory granules and transported to the neurohypophysis in axons that constitute the hypothalamo-hypophyseal tract. The hormones are released into fenestrated blood capillaries.

358. SUBJECT AREA: Endocrine System
QUESTION: The posterior pituitary

A: is composed of dense connective tissue.
B: has a portal blood supply.
C: contains pituicytes, Herring bodies and axons.
D: hormones that are glycoproteins.
E: exhibits all of the above features.

Learning Response C: Correct. The posterior pituitary or neurohypophysis consists of neuronal tissue: axons and glial cells. The glial cells are called pituicytes. The axon terminals are dilated with secretory product and are called Herring bodies. The adenohypophysis has a portal blood supply.

---

359. SUBJECT AREA: Endocrine System

QUESTION: In which region of the hypophysis would you expect to find the cells depicted in the figure below?

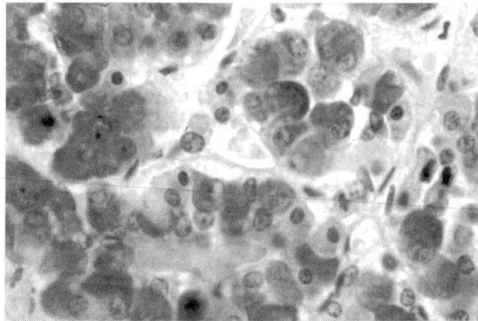

A: infundibular stalk
B: pars nervosa
C: pars intermedia
D: pars distalis
E: all of the above regions

Learning Response D: Correct. The micrograph depicts cells from the pars distalis of the adenohypophysis. The infundibular stalk and pars nervosa constitute the neurohypophysis which does not contain hormone secreting cells. The pars intermedia contains cords of cells with small secretory granules and obscure function.

360. SUBJECT AREA Endocrine System

QUESTION: Endocrine cells have all of the following anatomical distributions, except that they are NOT

A: a specialized gland.
B: clusters of cells in a gland.
C: individual cells dispersed among another cell type.
D: fascicles of cells in a gland.
E: blood-borne.

Learning Response E: Correct. Blood-borne cells that secrete cytokines/lymphokines are immunocytes (lymphocytes, macrophages or monocytes) and not considered classical endocrine cells. Examples: the thyroid is a specialized gland; the islets of Langerhans are clusters of cells within the pancreas; individual gastrin cells are dispersed throughout the intestine; some adrenocortical cells are aligned in fascicles in the zona fasciculata.

361. SUBJECT AREA: Endocrine System

QUESTION: All of the following are forms of endocrine mechanisms of control EXCEPT

A: autocrine secretion.
B: gap junctional communication.
C: paracrine secretion.
D: blood-borne transmission.
E: synaptic transmission.

Learning Response B: Correct. All the other mechanisms are common in the endocrine system. However, gap junctional communication requires neither secretion of a product (e.g., protein, peptide, steroid) nor receptor interaction. Neuroendocrine cells can secrete their hormone via synapses.

362. SUBJECT AREA: Endocrine System

QUESTION: Which of the following CANNOT be identified by granular morphology?

A: islet β cell
B: adrenomedullary cell
C: asymmetric synapse
D: adrenocortical cell
E: eosinophil

Learning Response D: Correct. Steroid secreting cells do not have a readily releasable pool of hormone; rather they synthesize steroid upon demand. This explains the lag in the rise of plasma cortisol compared to ACTH.

363. SUBJECT AREA: Endocrine System
        QUESTION: Steroid hormone receptors

A: are coupled to G-proteins.
B: are ion-gated channels.
C: are intracellular.
D: are intramembranous.
E: interact with carrier proteins on the cell membrane.

Learning Response C: Correct. These receptors can be in either the cytoplasm or the nucleus.

364. SUBJECT AREA: Endocrine System
        QUESTION: ACTH affects all of the following adrenal functions EXCEPT

A: aldosterone secretion.
B: norepinephrine conversion to epinephrine.
C: release of mineralocorticoids.
D: dehydroepiandrosterone secretion from the zona fasciculata.
E: cortisol release from the zona reticularis.

Learning Response B: Correct. ACTH affects the cortical steroid-producing cells. Adrenomedullary cells which secrete catecholamines are under control of the sympathetic nervous system.

365. SUBJECT AREA: Endocrine System
QUESTION: Mineralocorticoids

A: are primarily synthesized in the adrenal zona fasciculata.
B: stimulate sodium absorption by renal proximal convoluted tubules.
C: are involved in the maintenance of electrolytic balance.
D: activate the immune system.
E: are secreted in response to elevated blood glucocorticoid levels.

Learning Response C: Correct. Aldosterone acts on renal distal convoluted tubules to increase sodium absorption and facilitate the elimination of potassium and hydrogen ions.

366. SUBJECT AREA: Endocrine System
QUESTION: Glucocorticoids

A: have a catabolic effect on the liver.
B: suppress the immune response through inhibition of lymphocytic proliferation.
C: circulate back to the pituitary to stimulate the release of ACTH.
D: increase the synthetic activity of adipocytes.
E: affect blood glucose levels by inhibiting islet beta cells.

Learning Response B: Correct. This is a major factor in the immunosuppressive effect of cortisol. Glucocorticoids inhibit the release of ACTH from pituitary corticotrophs.

367. SUBJECT AREA: Endocrine System
QUESTION: All of the following are characteristics of an
adrenocortical cell EXCEPT

A: large amounts of smooth endoplasmic reticulum.
B: steroid-containing secretory granules.
C: vacuolated appearance at light microscopic level.
D: multiple mitochondria.
E: high lipid content.

Learning Response B: Correct. Steroid is not stored as a readily releasable
pool, but must be synthesized in response to a stimulus; this is why plasma
cortisol levels do not rise until 30–60 minutes after stimulation, whereas
plasma ACTH levels rise within 3 min.

368. SUBJECT AREA: Endocrine System
QUESTION: The fetal adrenal cortex

A: secretes mineralocorticoid.
B: differentiates into the adult zona fasciculata.
C: functions in the secretion of active androgens and
estrogens.
D: involutes at puberty.
E: converts into the adult sized gland through
hyperplasia.

Learning Response E: Correct. The permanent cortex is present in the fetus
as a very thin layer. The fetal cortex secretes sulfated conjugates of androgens
which are converted in the placenta to active androgens and estrogens.

369. SUBJECT AREA: Endocrine System
QUESTION: Chromaffin cells

A: receive synaptic input from postganglionic
parasympathetic fibers.
B: are 80% epinephrinergic.

C: can be differentiated from each other by their chromogranin content.

D: make catecholamines on demand rather than store it in secretory granules.

E: use dopamine-beta-hydroxylase to convert dopamine to L-dopa.

Learning Response B: Correct. Adrenomedullary chromaffin cells are modified sympathetic postganglionic cells, receiving input from presynaptic sympathetic neurons. Chromogranin is a common component of the secretory granules of both norepinephrinergic and epinephrinergic cells.

---

370. SUBJECT AREA: Endocrine System

QUESTION: All of the following are characteristics of the adrenal insufficiency in Addison's disease EXCEPT

A: an autoimmune disorder is involved.

B: 80% of the adrenal cortex is destroyed.

C: hypersecretion of glucocorticoids occurs.

D: a lack of secretion of mineralocorticoids occurs.

E: it is a complication of tuberculosis.

Learning Response C: Correct. Adrenal insufficiency would not result in hypersecretion.

---

371. SUBJECT AREA: Endocrine System

QUESTION: Hyperfunction of the adrenal with excessive glucocorticoid production (Cushing's syndrome)

A: is frequently due to adrenal hyperplasia.

B: is most often the result of a pituitary corticotrope adenoma.

C: is due to a lack of inhibitory feedback from the adrenal to pituitary.

D: also results in excessive aldosterone production.

E: is due to an adrenomedullary tumor.

Learning Response B: Correct. Rarely does adrenal hyperfunction involve both glucocorticoids and mineralocorticoids.

---

372. SUBJECT AREA: Endocrine System
QUESTION: Which of the following would NOT be found in adrenal chromaffin cells?

   A: prepronorepinephrine
   B: dopamine
   C: enkephalin
   D: prochromagranin
   E: tyrosine hydroxylase

Learning Response A: Correct. Norepinephrine is enzymatically converted from dopamine, rather than synthesized as a prohormone. Enzymatic pathway: tyrosine > dopa > dopamine > norepinephrine > epinephrine.

---

373. SUBJECT AREA: Endocrine System
QUESTION: Thyroid cells are different from most endocrine cells in that they

   A: have no secretory granules.
   B: store their product in the extracellular space.
   C: are actively engaged in pinocytosis.
   D: respond to a specific pituitary hormone.
   E: have abundant rough endoplasmic reticulum.

Learning Response B: Correct. Thyroid follicles are actually extracellular storage compartments for colloid (thyroglobulin).

---

374. SUBJECT AREA: Endocrine System
QUESTION: Parafollicular ("C") cells

   A: often reside inside the basal lamina of the thyroid epithelium.
   B: respond to thyroid stimulating hormone (TSH).
   C: are involved in the uptake of thyroglobulin.

D: have a typical steroid cell morphology.

E: supply carbohydrates for the glycosylation of thyroglobulin.

Learning Response A: Correct. Parafollicular cells are members of the DNES (diffuse neuroendocrine system), secrete a peptide hormone and do not directly participate in thyroid physiology.

375. SUBJECT AREA: Endocrine System

QUESTION: Parathyroid hormone (PTH) does all of the following EXCEPT

A: increase the activity of osteoclasts.

B: increase calcium levels in the blood.

C: reduce calcitonin secretion by parafollicular cells.

D: decrease phosphate absorption by kidney tubules.

E: increase absorption of calcium from the gastrointestinal tract.

Learning Response C: Correct. While PTH and calcitonin have opposing effects on blood calcium levels, PTH does not directly act on "C" cells.

376. SUBJECT AREA: Endocrine System

QUESTION: The secretion of parathyroid cells is regulated primarily by

A: blood calcium levels.

B: cholinergic input.

C: adrenergic input.

D: calcitonin levels.

E: thyroid stimulating hormone (TSH).

Learning Response A: Correct. PTH responds directly and rapidly to blood calcium levels.

377. SUBJECT AREA: Endocrine System
QUESTION: In the pineal gland,

        A: pinealocytes are a subtype of glial cell.
        B: serotonin is secreted by pinealocytes.
        C: oxyphil cells secrete melatonin.
        D: melatonin is stored in follicles in response to
           sympathetic input.
        E: astroglial cells store melatonin.

Learning Response B: Correct. Pinealocytes, the endocrine cells of the pineal gland, secrete melatonin and serotonin from secretory granules.

378. SUBJECT AREA: Endocrine System
QUESTION: Adrenocortical stimulation

        A: involves only glucocorticoid secretion.
        B: results in the exocytosis of steroid hormone
           granules.
        C: relies on adrenomedullary input.
        D: is inhibited by a reduction in circulating ACTH.
        E: is inhibited by vasopressin.

Learning Response D: Correct. Synthesis and secretion of glucocorticoids, mineralocorticoids and dehydroepiandrosterone from the adrenal cortex occur in response to elevated levels of plasma ACTH; as ACTH levels drop, the stimulus for synthesis is decreased and secretion is reduced.

379. SUBJECT AREA: Endocrine System
QUESTION: Which of the following is NOT a correct inhibitory
feedback loop?

        A: Parathyroid chief cell > osteoclasts >
           hypercalcemia > parathyroid chief cell
        B: Hypothalamus > pituitary thyrotropes > thyroid
           follicular cells > elevated plasma T_3/T_4 > pituitary
           thyrotropes

C: Hypothalamus > pituitary corticotropes > adrenocortical zona fasciculata > elevated glucocorticoid > hypothalamic neurons

D: Hypothalamic gonadotropin releasing hormone neurons > pituitary luteinizing hormone > interstitial (Leydig) cells > testosterone >pituitary gonadotrophic cells

E: Parafollicular "C" cell > osteoclasts > hypercalcemia > parafollicular cell

Learning Response E: Correct. The function of parafollicular cells is the secretion of calcitonin to inhibit osteoclasts, thereby reducing circulating levels of calcium. Therefore, hypercalcemia (an elevation in blood calcium levels) would turn on "C" cells, rather than inhibiting further secretion.

---

380. SUBJECT AREA: Endocrine System
QUESTION: All of the following endocrine diseases have an immune component to the disorder EXCEPT

A: Hashimoto's disease (hypothyroidism).
B: type I insulin-dependent diabetes mellitus (hypoinsulinemia).
C: pheochromocytoma of adrenal medulla.
D: Grave's disease (hyperthyroidism).
E: Addison's disease (adrenocortical insufficiency).

Learning Response C: Correct. Adrenal medullary tumors do not usually have an immunological component.

---

381. SUBJECT AREA: Endocrine System
QUESTION: Iodotyrosine dehalogenase

A: is present in the thyroid colloid.
B: degrades thyroglobulin into T_3 and T_4.
C: iodinates tyrosine residues in thyroglobulin.
D: activates iodide to combine with thyroglobulin.
E: recycles di- and mono-iodotyrosine into tyrosine and iodine.

Learning Response E: Correct. T_3, T_4, monoiodotyrosine (MIT) and diiodotyrosine (DIT) are all enzymatically converted from thyroglobulin in lysosomes and released into the cytoplasm. T_3 and T_4 are secreted, but MIT and DIT are recycled by iodotyrosine dehalogenase into iodine and tyrosine. Therefore, the presence of MIT and/or DIT in circulation is an indication of a metabolic disorder involving this enzyme.

---

382. SUBJECT AREA: Endocrine System

QUESTION: An active thyroid gland can be identified by all of the following EXCEPT

A: presence of columnar epithelial cells.
B: crenated colloid.
C: an increase in lysosomal activity.
D: an increase in the number of parafollicular cells.
E: reduced follicular size.

Learning Response D: Correct. Thyroid and parafollicular activities are independent of each other. The follicle is a storage compartment that should shrink as thyroglobulin is utilized by the active gland.

---

383. SUBJECT AREA: Endocrine System

QUESTION: Each of the following pairs have opposing actions EXCEPT

A: parafollicular cell calcitonin : chief cell parathyroid hormone.
B: islet alpha cell glucagon : islet beta cell insulin.
C: hypothalamic somatostatin : hypophythalamic growth hormone releasing hormone.
D: hypothalamic corticotropin releasing hormone : adrenocortical cortisol.
E: posterior pituitary antidiuretic hormone (ADH) : adrenocortical aldosterone.

Learning Response E: Correct. ADH acts by making renal collecting ducts permeable to water (water balance); aldosterone acts on renal distal convoluted tubules to increase sodium absorption and eliminate potassium and hydrogen ions (osmotic balance). Calcitonin and PTH affect blood calcium levels; glucagon and insulin affect blood glucose levels; somatostatin and GnRH affect GH secretion; CRH and cortisol affect ACTH release.

---

384. SUBJECT AREA: Endocrine System

QUESTION: All of the following are morphologic changes that occur with age EXCEPT

A: calcium accumulation in the pineal gland.
B: involution of the thyroid follicles.
C: accumulation of lipofuscin in neurons.
D: involution of the thymus.
E: an increase in oxyphil cells in the parathyroids.

Learning Response B: Correct. The thyroid may become less active with age, causing a stasis in follicular size; however, the follicles do not actually involute The accumulation of radio-opaque calcium in the pineal gland is a convenient radiologic landmark for the midline in a brain scan.

---

385. SUBJECT AREA: Endocrine System

QUESTION: Fenestrated capillaries are present in all of the following regions EXCEPT

A: hypothalamic median eminence.
B: adrenal cortex.
C: islets of Langerhans.
D: pancreatic lobules.
E: choroid plexus.

Learning Response D: Correct. Fenestrated capillaries are common in endocrine organs.

---

386. SUBJECT AREA: Endocrine System

QUESTION: The dominant cell type in the figure below has the morphologic characteristics of a cell that

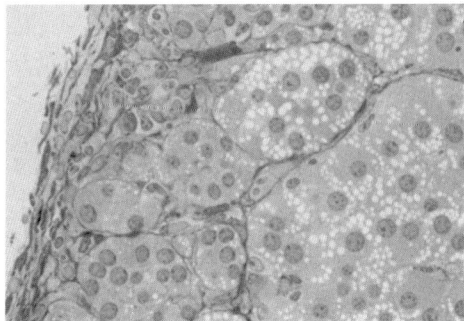

A: stores large amounts of glycogen.
B: contains many lipid droplets.
C: is packed with smooth endoplasmic reticulum.
D: contains a translucent product in secretory granules.
E: is poorly fixed due to a relatively impenetrable membrane.

Learning Response B: Correct. Standard preparatory steps for tissue light microscopy use solvents that dissolve lipid, resulting in a moth-eaten appearance of cells with many lipid droplets, such as these steroid-producing cells of the adrenocortical zona fasciculata. The same effect can be seen in multilocular adipose tissue.

387. SUBJECT AREA: Endocrine System
QUESTION: In which region of the adrenal gland would you expect to find the type of cell pictured in the figure below?

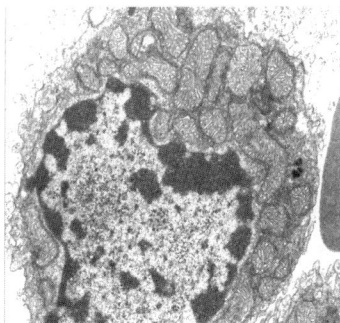

A: capsule
B: zona glomerulosa
C: zona fasciculata
D: zona reticularis
E: medulla

Learning Response B: Correct. The cells of the zona glomerulosa contain an abundance of mitochondria with shelf cristae. The mitochondria of cells in the inner two zones of the cortex have tubular cristae. The capsule and medulla lack cells with an abundance of mitochondria and lipid typical of the cells of the cortex.

---

388. SUBJECT AREA: Endocrine System
QUESTION: Thyroid colloid is composed of high molecular weight

A: cholesterol molecules.
B: lipoprotein.
C: polysaccharide.
D: nucleic acid.
E: glycoprotein.

Learning Response E: Correct. The secretory product of the follicular cells is stored in the extracellular colloid bound to a glycoprotein until it is taken back into the cells. At that time, the peptide bonds between the iodinated residues and thyroglobulin are cleaved by proteases and the hormonal products are released into the blood stream.

---

389. SUBJECT AREA: Endocrine System
QUESTION: The D cell, or delta cell, of the endocrine pancreas produces

A: insulin.
B: pancreatic polypeptide.
C: somatotropin.
D: somatostatin.
E: pancreozymin.

Learning Response D: Correct. Insulin and glucagon are secreted by islet beta and alpha cells, respectively. Pancreatic polypeptide is produced by islet F cells. Somatotropin or growth hormone is released from the pituitary, and pancreozymin is a synonym for cholecystokinin or CCK which stimulates the exocrine pancreas.

390. SUBJECT AREA: Digestive System
QUESTION: Which of the following are secretions of gastric parietal cells?

    A: hydrochloric acid
    B: pepsinogen
    C: gastric intrinsic factor
    D: Choices A and B above
    E: Choices A and C above

Learning Response E: Correct. Gastric parietal cells secrete hydrochloric acid and intrinsic factor. They also secrete bicarbonate ions into the gastric interstitial tissue. The chief cells synthesize and secrete pepsinogen.

391. SUBJECT AREA: Digestive System
QUESTION: Which of the following structures is ABSENT from the ileum?

    A: submucosal glands
    B: Paneth cells
    C: goblet cells
    D: Peyer's patches
    E: villi

Learning Response A: Correct. Brunner's glands are mucus secreting glands in the submucosa of the duodenum, and are absent from the ileum. All of the other choices are components of the ileum.

392. SUBJECT AREA: Digestive System
QUESTION: Teniae coli form which of the following layers of the colon?

A: muscularis mucosa
B: lamina propria
C: submucosa
D: outer layer of muscularis externa
E: inner layer of muscularis externa

Learning Response D: Correct. The smooth muscle fibers of the outer longitudinal layer of the colon are arranged into three thick bands called teniae coli.

393. SUBJECT AREA: Digestive System
QUESTION: Identify the only type of lingual papillae that does NOT usually possess taste buds.

A: filiform
B: fungiform
C: circumvallate
D: foliate

Learning Response A: Correct. Taste buds can be found on all of the lingual papillae except filiform papillae which are the most numerous. Filiform papillae are present over the entire surface of the tongue and their epithelium may be at least partially keratinized.

394. SUBJECT AREA: Digestive System
QUESTION: In the gastrointestinal tract,

A: Paneth cells located at the base of the intestinal crypts secrete bacteriocidal agents.
B: the region of the esophagus near its junction with the stomach usually lacks glandular components.
C: the principal site of stem cell proliferation is at the base of the gastric glands.
D: the majority of cells in the cardiac and pyloric portions of the stomach produce immunoglobulins.
E: parasympathetic neurons in the submucosal plexus (of Meissner) send axons to the muscularis externa.

Learning Response A: Correct. Paneth cells in the crypts of the small intestine produce lysozyme which hydrolyzes bacterial cell walls. The esophagus near the junction with the stomach contains mucus secreting glands in the mucosa and submucosa. Stem cell proliferation in the stomach occurs at the entrance to the gastric glands in the neck mucous cells. The cells in the cardiac and pyloric epithelia are mucus secreting cells. The parasympathetic neurons of the submucosal plexus innervate the smooth muscle cells in the muscularis mucosae.

---

395. SUBJECT AREA: Digestive System

QUESTION: All of the following are characteristic of the cells of the diffuse neuroendocrine system EXCEPT

A: their polarity is opposite to that of gastric chief cells.

B: they may extend from the lumen to the basal lamina of the intestinal epithelium.

C: their production of gastrin increases acid production by parietal cells.

D: they empty their contents directly into the lumen of the gland.

E: they can secrete hormones which can interact with neighboring cells.

Learning Response D: Correct. The neuroendocrine cells of the gastrointestinal tract secrete the hormones into the interstitial space From there the products enter the blood stream.

---

396. SUBJECT AREA: Digestive System

QUESTION: In gut associated lymphoid tissue (GALT),

A: IgA produced by plasma cells is transported by the enterocytes to attack bacteria in the intercellular space.

B: M cells synthesize and secrete antibodies.

C: B lymphocytes that are activated in the gut wall may proliferate in lymph nodes distant from the alimentary canal.

D: lymphoid nodules are rarely found in the
   connective tissue of the small intestine.
E: lymphocytes are excluded from the intestinal
   epithelium.

Learning Response C: Correct. M cells function as antigen presenting cells
which activate intraepithelial lymphocytes, some of which can migrate from
the intestinal connective tissue and populate lymph nodes distant from the
initial activation site. Plasma cells in the lamina propria secrete IgA which is
taken up by the enterocytes and transported to the lumen where it attaches to
antigenic sites on gut bacteria. Lymphoid nodules are often located in the gut
wall, especially in the ileum where aggregated nodules constitute Peyer's
patches.

---

397. SUBJECT AREA: Digestive System
            QUESTION: All of the following may occur after surgical removal
                      of the stomach EXCEPT

A: vitamin B_{12} absorption in the intestine would most
   likely be affected by the loss of parietal cells.
B: the body's total population of gastrin secreting cells
   would be lost.
C: the presence of D cells (somatostatin secreting
   cells) in other areas of the intestinal tract would
   compensate for the loss of gastric D cells.
D: the levels of pepsinogen and rennin would decline
   as a result of the loss of gastric chief cells.
E: the source of intrinsic factor would be lost.

Learning Response B: Correct. The stomach is not the only source of gastrin
secreting cells. These cells can also be found in the proximal regions of the
small intestine.

---

398. SUBJECT AREA: Digestive System
            QUESTION: In the stomach,

A: chief cells are rich in apical secretory granules
   which are positive for lysozyme.

B: the base of the gastric glands is the principal site of stem cell associated proliferation.

C: the glycoproteins secreted by surface and neck mucous cells protect the gastric epithelium from proteolytic action.

D: bicarbonate secretion by parietal cells during acid secretion protects the interstitium from high pH.

E: chief and parietal cells can be found in the cardiac, main body and pyloric regions.

Learning Response C: Correct. Chief and parietal cells are restricted to the fundus and main body of the stomach and are essentially absent from the uppermost and lowermost regions. Chief cells secrete proteolytic enzymes, especially pepsinogen, gastric lipase and rennin; the latter is important for the digestion of milk proteins. Lysozyme is produced by mucus secreting cells in the cardia and pylorus. Bicarbonate ions in the interstitium protect that region from any leakage of the low pH material from the lumen. The main site of stem cell proliferation is the neck or apical area of the gastric glands.

399. SUBJECT AREA: Digestive System

QUESTION: The villus-crypt unit

A: is a distinguishing feature of the colon.

B: may contain Paneth cells which secrete lysozyme.

C: contains cells which arise from stem cells in the villus tip and migrate to the crypt.

D: has a ratio of villus length to crypt length which is constant throughout the gastrointestinal tract.

E: does not contain glandular components.

Learning Response B: Correct. Although the crypts are part of the mucosa of the large intestine, villi are absent there. The stem cells of the villus-crypt unit are located in the crypt and migrate to the tip of the villus where they are shed. The ratio of villus length to crypt length varies in the small intestine. The jejunum has the tallest villi of the three regions of the small intestine.

400. SUBJECT AREA: Digestive System

QUESTION: Histological features of the appendix include

A: an abundance of lymphoid nodules.
B: the absence of tenia coli.
C: the absence of villi.
D: the presence of goblet cells.
E: all of the above characteristics.

Learning Response E: Correct. The appendix is similar in structure to the large intestine, but it contains a number of lymphoid nodules in its wall which help to distinguish it from the colon.

401. SUBJECT AREA: Digestive System
QUESTION: The apical surface of absorptive cells or enterocytes (including the glycocalyx) is specialized to

A: protect against bacterial infection.
B: digest dipeptides.
C: adsorb polypeptides.
D: transport triglycerides.
E: absorb polysaccharides.

Learning Response B: Correct. Among the functions of the enterocytes is the digestion of small dipeptides and disaccharides by enzymes located in the glycocalyx. The enterocytes absorb amino acids and monosaccharides. Paneth cells secrete bacteriocidal substances, and the immune system in the gut protects the region. The enterocytes absorb monoglycerides, glycerol and fatty acids from the lumen and resynthesize triglycerides intracellularly.

402. SUBJECT AREA: Digestive System
QUESTION: All of the following are characteristics of ameloblasts EXCEPT

A: tight junctions are located at both the apical and basal regions of the cells.
B: that they secrete procollagen which ultimately forms the dentin of developing teeth.
C: the presence of rough endoplasmic reticulum and a prominent Golgi complex indicate that they are capable of secreting proteins.

    D: the secretory activity of the cells is located
primarily at the cytoplasm adjacent to the basal
lamina.

    E: that they function in the destruction of the basal
lamina separating ameloblasts from odontoblasts.

Learning Response B: Correct. Ameloblasts are epithelial cells in that they secrete material into the basal lamina. In addition to removing the basal lamina between them and odontoblasts, ameloblasts secrete the organic matrix of enamel. Odontoblasts are responsible for the formation of dentin from procollagen which they synthesize and secrete.

---

403. SUBJECT AREA: Digestive System

    QUESTION: All of the following are features of the oral mucosa
EXCEPT that it

    A: contains Langerhans' cells.

    B: has layers similar to those found in thin skin.

    C: is not tightly adherent to the underlying lamina
propria on the hard palate.

    D: is lined by nonkeratinized stratified squamous
epithelium.

    E: is thin enough in some areas to allow the
absorption of drugs into the circulatory system.

Learning Response C: Correct. The oral mucosa is tightly adherent to the lamina propria of the hard palate which is in contact with bony tissue. Since the oral mucosa has characteristics similar to that of thin skin, all of the other statements are true of this structure.

---

404. SUBJECT AREA: Digestive System

    QUESTION: The lining cells of the stomach produce

    A: pepsinogen.

    B: mucus.

    C: rennin.

    D: gastrin.

    E: renin.

Learning Response B: Correct. The surface cells of the stomach produce a viscous mucus which protects the underlying cells from the acidic environment of the lumen. Pepsinogen and rennin are synthesized by the gastric chief cells, and gastrin is produced by the cells of the diffuse neuroendocrine system. Renin is secreted by the juxtaglomerular cells of the kidney.

405. SUBJECT AREA: Digestive System
QUESTION: The duodenum

A: is lined by ciliated simple columnar epithelium.
B: contains aggregated lymphoid nodules called Peyer's patches.
C: does not exhibit villi.
D: contains mucus secreting glands in the submucosa.
E: lacks an external longitudinal smooth muscle layer.

Learning Response D: Correct. Mucus secreting glands (also known as Brunner's glands) are located in the submucosa of the duodenum. The organ is lined with simple columnar epithelium which has a brush border. Other features of the duodenum include the presence of villi and an external longitudinal muscle coat. Peyer's patches are found in the ileum.

406. SUBJECT AREA: Digestive System
QUESTION: Lacteals

A: transport glucose.
B: are lymphatic capillaries.
C: breakdown milk proteins.
D: transport pancreatic hormones.
E: are venous sinusoids in the lamina propria.

Learning Response B: Correct. Lymphatic capillaries in the lamina propria of the villi are lacteals which transport the products of the digestion of lipids (chylomicrons).

407. SUBJECT AREA: Digestive System
QUESTION: The tongue

A: is primarily composed of smooth muscle.

B: is completely covered with a keratinized epithelium.

C: contains minor salivary glands which secrete lipase.

D: has several differently shaped papillae all of which have taste buds.

E: is one of the regions of the oral cavity which lacks lymphoid tissue.

Learning Response C: Correct. Von Ebner's glands are minor salivary glands associated with the tongue, and the cells of these glands secrete a lipase which prevents the formation of a hydrophobic layer over the taste buds. Partial keratinization occurs over the filiform papillae which lack taste buds. The lingual tonsils are aggregations of lymphoid tissue located in the posterior region of the tongue.

408. SUBJECT AREA: Digestive System

QUESTION: Arrange the following structures in correct sequence from lumen to external wall.

A: adventitia, mucosa, submucosa, serosa

B: serosa, mucosa, submucosa, muscularis mucosae

C: mucosa, submucosa, muscularis mucosae, serosa

D: mucosa, submucosa, muscularis externa, adventitia

E: muscularis mucosae, submucosa, serosa, muscularis externa

Learning Response D: Correct. The general organization of the digestive tract consists of a inner lining mucosa, which is composed of an epithelial layer, an underlying connective tissue layer (lamina propria) and a muscularis mucosae. Beneath the mucosa is the submucosa, which is composed of connective tissue and may contain glands. Adjacent to the submucosa is the muscularis externa, which usually has two layers of smooth muscle. The outermost layer of the wall consists of either a serosa, which is a thin connective tissue layer covered by simple squamous epithelium, or an adventitia, which is the connective tissue of the body wall covering the organs not invested with peritoneum.

409. SUBJECT AREA: Digestive System
QUESTION: In the teeth,

A: dentin is external to the enamel layer.
B: type III collagen forms the major protein component of both dentin and enamel.
C: enamel extends beneath the gingiva to cover the root.
D: the periodontal ligament serves as the periosteum of the alveolar bone.
E: unlike enamel which is rich in calcium, dentin lacks a calcified component.

Learning Response D: Correct. Along the root of the tooth, the collagenous periodontal ligament anchors the tooth to alveolar bone and can be considered to be the periosteum of the bone socket. Enamel is the external layer of the crown of the tooth, and dentin lies beneath it. Dentin extends into the root which is capped by a layer of cementum, which is similar to bone. Type I collagen is found in dentin which is also a calcified tissue.

410. SUBJECT AREA: Digestive System
QUESTION: All of the following are features of the esophagus EXCEPT

A: the presence of smooth muscle cells in the upper third of the organ.
B: mucus secreting esophageal glands in the submucosa.
C: mucus secreting glands in the lamina propria in the region closest to the stomach.
D: the presence of a lining of nonkeratinized stratified squamous epithelium.
E: the majority of the organ is covered by adventitia.

Learning Response A: Correct. The upper part of the esophagus has striated muscle in its external muscle layer, and the lowermost region, smooth muscle. The middle third of the organ contains a mixture of striated and smooth muscle cells.

411. SUBJECT AREA: Digestive System
QUESTION: The absorptive surface of the small intestine is increased by the presence of all of the following EXCEPT

A: microvilli.
B: plicae circulares.
C: villi.
D: external folds.
E: rugae.

Learning Response E: Correct. Rugae are impermanent, longitudinal folds of the mucosa and submucosa of the stomach. All of the other structures add to the surface area of the small intestine.

412. SUBJECT AREA: Digestive System
QUESTION: Innervation of the digestive tract occurs via neurons associated with

A: the myenteric plexus (of Auerbach).
B: the submucosal plexus (of Meissner).
C: the sympathetic ganglia.
D: the parasympathetic system.
E: all of the above choices.

Learning Response E: Correct. The gastrointestinal tract is innervated by extrinsic components which are part of the sympathetic and parasympathetic nervous systems and by intrinsic components within the myenteric and submucosal plexuses.

413. SUBJECT AREA: Digestive System
QUESTION: In the figure below, the core of the structures shown here consists primarily of

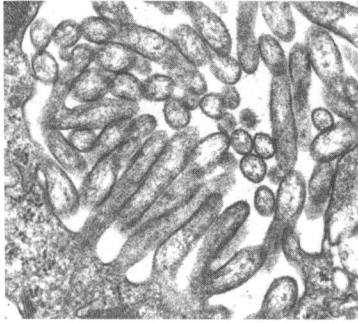

A: microtubules.
B: actin microfilaments.
C: intermediate filaments.
D: type III collagen.
E: tonofilaments.

Learning Response B: Correct. Actin filaments within the microvilli are enclosed by the plasmalemma and its glycocalyx. Microtubules and intermediate filaments (tonofilaments) may be found within the cytoplasm of the cell, but are never within microvilli. Collagen is always located extracellularly.

414. SUBJECT AREA: Digestive System
       QUESTION: Identify the type of cell marked by the arrowhead in the figure below.

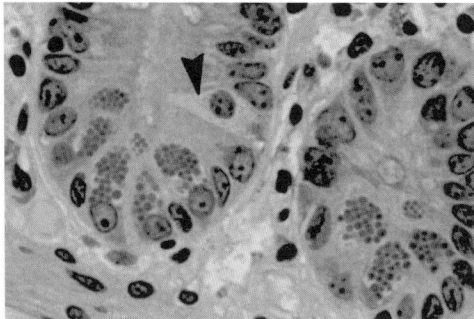

A: absorptive epithelial cell
B: gastric chief cell
C: enteroendocrine cell

D: Paneth cell
E: goblet cell

Learning Response C: Correct. The cell extends from the lumen at the upper left to the basement membrane. Secretory granules would be found in its cytoplasm near the basal connective tissue, indicating that the cell deposits its products into the underlying connective tissue. Therefore, this cell is part of the diffuse neuroendocrine system, an enteroendocrine cell, of the open type.

---

415. SUBJECT AREA: Digestive System
QUESTION: Identify the organ shown in the figure below.

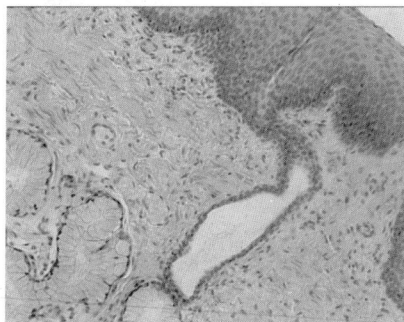

A: esophagus
B: large intestine
C: rectum
D: anus
E: stomach

Learning Response A: Correct. The esophagus is lined by nonkeratinized stratified squamous epithelium, and contains mucous glands in the submucosa. All of the other structures listed above, with the exception of the anus, are lined by columnar epithelium. The anal canal lacks submucosal glands.

---

416. SUBJECT AREA: Digestive System
QUESTION: What is the function of the cell shown in the figure below?

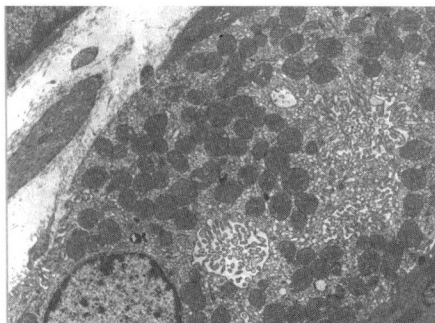

A: production of intrinsic factor
B: production of digestive enzymes
C: production of hydrogen ions
D: choices A and B above
E: choices A and C above

Learning Response E: Correct. The image depicts a parietal cell from the gastric mucosa which produces hydrogen ions which contribute to the acid milieu of the lumen and intrinsic factor which aids the intestine in the absorption of vitamin B_{12}. Persons deficient in this vitamin can have a disease of the erythrocytes called pernicious anemia.

417. SUBJECT AREA: Digestive System
QUESTION: Identify the type of cell that contains the large secretory granules as depicted in the figure below.

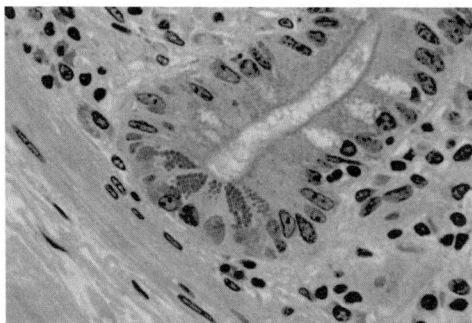

A: gastric chief cell
B: enteroendocrine cell
C: goblet cell

D: Paneth cell
E: myoepithelial cell

Learning Response D: Correct. Located at the base of the intestinal crypts, Paneth cells contain secretory granules of lysozyme, an important bacteriocidal agent. Gastric chief cells have numerous secretory granules which are much smaller in diameter than those of Paneth cells. The presence of goblet cells indicates that the organ is not the stomach.

---

418. SUBJECT AREA: Glands of the Digestive System
QUESTION: The lining of bile canaliculi consists of

A: simple cuboidal epithelium.
B: simple squamous epithelium.
C: simple columnar epithelium.
D: the plasma membrane of Kupffer cells.
E: the plasma membranes of adjacent hepatocytes.

Learning Response E: Correct. Electron microscopy has shown that adjacent hepatocytes form the bile canaliculi. Tight junctions between the hepatocytes seal the lumen of the channels and prevent leakage of bile into the intercellular space.

---

419. SUBJECT AREA: Glands of the Digestive System
QUESTION: The major function of the gall bladder is to

A: transport bile.
B: synthesize bile.
C: concentrate bile.
D: break down bile.
E: secrete enzymes.

Learning Response C: Correct. The main function of the gall bladder is to store bile and to concentrate it by absorbing water. Bile, which is synthesized in the liver, is released into the digestive tract in response to cholecystokinin.

420. SUBJECT AREA: Glands of the Digestive System
QUESTION: In the liver,

A: the hepatocytes produce bile which is secreted into a duct system lined by columnar epithelia.
B: venous and arterial blood mix in the sinusoids.
C: the sinusoidal epithelium is continuous to prevent exposure of hepatocytes to bacterial toxins.
D: hepatocytes are joined on two sides by tight junctions to prevent the passage of plasma between cells in a cord of hepatocytes.
E: bile and blood flow in the same direction.

Learning Response B: Correct. The hepatic sinusoids which are large caliber, discontinuous capillaries contain a mixture of blood from branches of the hepatic artery and portal vein. Bile produced by the hepatocytes is deposited in the bile canaliculi which are channels lined by the plasmalemma of the hepatocytes. Bile flows in a direction opposite to that of blood. The endothelium of the sinusoids has large gaps in its wall to facilitate the passage of macromolecules to and from the hepatocytes.

421. SUBJECT AREA: Glands of the Digestive System
QUESTION: In comparing the parotid gland with the pancreas,

A: striated ducts are found in both glands.
B: intercalated ducts are found in the pancreas and absent from the parotid.
C: centroacinar cells are found in both glands.
D: both glands function in the synthesis and secretion of digestive enzymes.
E: both glands have clusters of hormone secreting cells.

Learning Response D: Correct. The parotid glands secrete salivary amylase and the pancreas secretes a variety of digestive enzymes. Striated ducts are located in the parotid gland and not in the pancreas. Intercalated ducts are found in both, and centroacinar cells are restricted to the pancreas which has clusters of hormone secreting cells constituting the islets of Langerhans.

422. SUBJECT AREA: Glands of the Digestive System
QUESTION: In reference to the liver,

A: blood and bile flow in the same direction in the hepatic acinus.

B: a single type of cell is responsible for bilirubin modification, vitamin A storage, drug detoxification, cholesterol synthesis and phagocytosis of effete blood cells.

C: the portal vein delivers deoxygenated blood to the hepatic sinusoids from the alimentary canal, spleen and pancreas.

D: the bile canaliculi drain into the portal veins in the portal triads.

E: the hepatocytes break down bile into its components of bile salts, phospholipids, cholesterol and pigments.

Learning Response C: Correct. The portal vein is rich in nutrients from the alimentary canal and also drains the spleen and pancreas. The poorly oxygenated blood is delivered to the sinusoids via branches of the portal vein. In the acinus, as in the classical and portal lobule concepts, blood and bile flow in opposite directions: blood away from the portal triads, bile toward that region. Several different types of cells are responsible for the diverse functions of the liver: hepatocytes, fat storing cells and phagocytic cells (Kupffer cells).

423. SUBJECT AREA: Glands of the Digestive System
QUESTION: In reference to the pancreas,

A: digestive enzymes are constitutively secreted.

B: the centroacinar cells secrete enzymes which are activated in the duodenum.

C: duct cells secrete bicarbonate which will neutralize the acidity of chyme entering the duodenum from the stomach.

D: a depletion of the cells that secrete cholecystokinin (CCK) will have no effect on the acinar cells.

E: increased levels of blood glucose will cause the

alpha cells to secrete increased amounts of
glucagon.

Learning Response C: Correct. Secretin promotes the secretion of bicarbonate
ions which neutralize the acidity of chyme from the stomach. The acinar cells
produce digestive enzymes in response to cholecystokinin and, thus, the
enzymes are not constitutively secreted but are regulated by the hormone The
centroacinar cells do not secrete digestive enzymes, and the beta cells of the
islets respond to increased blood glucose levels.

424. SUBJECT AREA: Glands of the Digestive System
QUESTION: All of the following are characteristic of the salivary
glands EXCEPT

A: myoepithelial cells are located within the basal
lamina of the duct cells.
B: the smallest diameter ducts are the intercalated
ducts.
C: most of the acini of the sublingual glands are
serous acini.
D: connective tissue plasma cells secrete IgA, a
component of immune reactions in the oral cavity.
E: the parotid gland consists mainly of serous acini.

Learning Response C: Correct. The sublingual gland contains a mixture of
mucous and serous acini, and the mucous acini predominate The remainder
of the above selections are true of the salivary glands.

425. SUBJECT AREA: Glands of the Digestive System
QUESTION: In the pancreas,

A: the endocrine and exocrine portions of the gland
are integrated within each secretory acinus.
B: the centroacinar cell is the first cell of the duct
system.
C: interlobular ducts are absent.
D: glucagon is localized in the delta cells of the islets.
E: the acinar cells secrete acid hydrolases which

function in digestion in the stomach.

Learning Response B: Correct. Centroacinar cells, which are the initial cells of the intercalated ducts, are characteristic of the pancreas. The endocrine and exocrine regions of the gland are separated from each other by connective tissue. Interlobular ducts are located in the connective tissue between the lobules. The acinar cells secrete enzymes which function in digestive processes in the duodenum. Glucagon is secreted by the alpha cells of the islets, insulin by the beta cells and somatostatin by the delta cells.

426. SUBJECT AREA: Glands of the Digestive System
QUESTION: Surgical removal of the gall bladder would most likely result in

A: no adverse effect on cholecystokinin (CCK) producing cells.
B: cessation of lipid absorption by the enterocytes.
C: an absence of chylomicrons in the portal vein.
D: cessation of bile secretion.
E: increased levels of bilirubin in the peripheral blood.

Learning Response A: Correct. The gall bladder stores and concentrates bile. CCK secreting cells are not located in the gall bladder, but are distributed widely in the mucosa of the small intestine Bile secretion and bilirubin excretion by hepatocytes would not be affected.

427. SUBJECT AREA: Glands of the Digestive System
QUESTION: What *specifically* distinguishes a hepatocyte from any other type of cell?

A: Abundant lysosomes
B: Synthesis of plasma proteins, especially albumin, fibrinogen and lipoproteins
C: Synthesis of bilirubin from heme
D: Prominent smooth endoplasmic reticulum (ER)
E: Presence of peroxisomes

Learning Response B: Correct. One of the major hepatic functions is the secretion of a number of different plasma proteins. An abundance of lysosomes would also be found in phagocytic cells, smooth ER in steroid-secreting cells, peroxisomes in cells of the kidney. Bilirubin synthesis occurs in the spleen, and the pigment is excreted in bile produced by the liver.

---

428. SUBJECT AREA: Glands of the Digestive System
QUESTION: In the pancreas,

A: digestive enzymes may be released from acinar cells upon stimulation by gastrin.
B: there are neuroendocrine cells that synthesize some of the digestive enzymes.
C: numerous mitochondria are a feature of centroacinar cells.
D: the cells producing insulin and glucagon can be distinguished on the basis of secretory granule morphology.
E: the basophilic portions of the acinar cells are located in the apical regions of the cells.

Learning Response D: Correct. The glucagon secreting cells have regularly shaped granules with a dense core and a clear region between the core and the membrane. Insulin secreting cells have irregular granules with a core of crystals of insulin coupled with zinc. Regulated secretion of digestive enzymes is controlled by cholecystokinin, and only acinar cells secrete digestive enzymes. Centroacinar cells have few mitochondria, and the basal regions of acinar cells contain stacks of rough endoplasmic reticulum contributing to the basophilia of that part of the cells.

---

429. SUBJECT AREA: Glands of the Digestive System
QUESTION: In the liver acinus, the hepatocytes in Zone I (the region closest to the portal canals)

A: would have the highest amounts of glycogen.
B: would have the highest exposure to toxins.
C: would have the highest exposure to nutrients.
D: would be expected to have the highest level of oxidative metabolism.

E: would exhibit all of the above features.

Learning Response E: Correct. The hepatocytes in Zone I of the acinus would have all of the features listed above.

---

430. SUBJECT AREA: Glands of the Digestive System
QUESTION: All of the following are true of hepatocytes EXCEPT that they

A: can function as both exocrine and endocrine cells.
B: take up IgA polymers from the plasma.
C: contain peroxisomes which function in fatty acid oxidation and hydrogen peroxide degradation.
D: contain variable amounts of glycogen associated with regions of smooth endoplasmic reticulum.
E: synthesize and secrete cholecystokinin (CCK) which acts on the gall bladder.

Learning Response E: Correct. Cells of the enteroendocrine system in the small intestine and elsewhere release CCK which stimulates the gall bladder to secrete bile and the pancreas to secrete digestive enzymes. The ability of hepatocytes to secrete bile which is eventually transported to a duct system identifies the exocrine function of the liver. Secretion of plasma proteins into the blood stream constitutes its endocrine function.

---

431. SUBJECT AREA: Glands of the Digestive System
QUESTION: In the oral cavity,

A: bacteriocidal agents are secreted by striated duct cells to protect the oral cavity from pathogens.
B: the largest salivary gland ducts found in the stromal tissue between the lobules are the secretory or intralobular ducts which are lined with columnar epithelium.
C: parasympathetic stimulation of the salivary glands elicits the production of a viscous fluid with little protein content.
D: the secretory product of the serous acinar cells of

the sublingual gland is more viscous than that of
the mucous acini.

E: striated duct cells of the parotid gland may modify
the composition of the secretion.

Learning Response E: Correct. The acinar cells, intercalated duct cells and
striated duct cells synthesize a secretory component which complexes with
immunoglobulin A to facilitate passage of the antibody through the epithelial
cells and into the salivary fluid. Acinar cells and intercalated duct cells also
produce lysozyme and lactoferrin which act to protect against pathogenic
bacteria. The large ducts of the salivary glands are the interlobular or
excretory ducts which are located in the connective tissue between the
lobules. Serous acinar cells produce a watery secretion while mucus secreting
acinar cells secrete a viscous fluid. Parasympathetic stimulation produces a
copious, watery salivary fluid which contains small amounts of organic
material.

432. SUBJECT AREA: Glands of the Digestive System
        QUESTION: In reference to the salivary glands,

A: the sublingual gland has many striated ducts so that
its mucous secretion can be modified.

B: the minor salivary glands of the oral mucosa are
mostly mucous glands.

C: myoepithelial cells surrounding salivary gland acini
are controlled by the autonomic nervous system.

D: intercalated ducts, the largest caliber intralobular
ducts, empty directly into the interlobular ducts.

E: a mixed salivary gland has serous acini with
mucous demilunes.

Learning Response C: Correct. Myoepithelial cells help to release the
products of the salivary gland cells into the duct system and are, thus,
controlled by the parasympathetic and sympathetic divisions of the autonomic
nervous system. Minor salivary glands such as von Ebner's glands in the
tongue are mainly composed of serous acini. The sublingual gland, which is a
mixed gland with mucous acini and serous demilunes, has few striated ducts,
and the intercalated ducts are the smallest of the intralobular ducts and empty
into the striated ducts.

433. SUBJECT AREA: Glands of the Digestive System

QUESTION: The primary function of the fat-storing cells associated with the perisinusoidal space (of Disse) is

A: the production of bilirubin.

B: in the immune reactions of the liver.

C: accumulation of vitamin A as retinyl esters in lipid droplets.

D: detoxification of exogenously delivered barbiturates.

E: synthesis and secretion of steroid hormones.

Learning Response C: Correct. Fat-storing cells have the capacity to store vitamin A in their lipid droplets. Hepatocytes carry out the detoxification reactions of the liver, and the phagocytic Kupffer cells are probably involved in hepatic immune responses. Bilirubin is produced in the spleen as the result of hemolysis of erythrocytes.

434. SUBJECT AREA: Glands of the Digestive System

QUESTION: The hepatocytes most severely affected by hypoxia (decreased oxygen levels) would be located

A: near the portal triad.

B: near the terminal hepatic venule (central vein).

C: in the center of a liver acinus.

D: in Zone II of the liver acinus.

E: adjacent to the connective tissue capsule.

Learning Response B: Correct. Oxygenated blood is delivered to the hepatic lobule by the hepatic artery and its tributaries within the portal triad. The cells farthest away from the triad area would be the most susceptible to reduced oxygen levels, and these cells would be located closest to the terminal hepatic venules. Zone II of the liver acinus is found part way between the triad and the central vein.

435. SUBJECT AREA: Glands of the Digestive System

QUESTION: Obstructive jaundice can occur from blockage of the common bile duct by gallstones that pass from the gall bladder. Such an obstruction in the common bile duct can result in

A: an accumulation of bile in the hepatic bile canaliculi.

B: an impaired breakdown of fats in the small intestine because of the lack of emulsifying bile acids.

C: an enlargement of the gall bladder resulting from the retention of bile.

D: a flattening of the mucosal folds of the gall bladder.

E: all of the above choices.

Learning Response E: Correct. It is probable that all of the events listed above would occur as a result of an obstruction of the common bile duct which is formed by the union of the hepatic duct and the cystic duct.

436. SUBJECT AREA: Glands of the Digestive System

QUESTION: All of the following are true of the perisinusoidal space (of Disse) EXCEPT

A: it is supported by type I collagen fibrils.

B: microvilli from the hepatocytes project into the space.

C: it is lined by both endothelial cells and phagocytic cells.

D: it permits contact of blood fluids with the hepatocytes.

E: macromolecules secreted by the hepatocytes first pass into the space.

Learning Response A: Correct. The perisinusoidal space is supported by delicate reticular fibers composed of type III collagen.

437. SUBJECT AREA: Glands of the Digestive System

QUESTION: The secretory acini depicted in the figure below would most likely be found in the

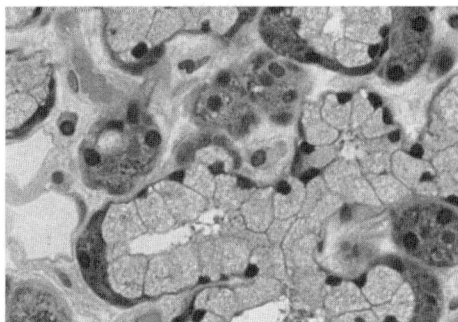

A: pancreas.
B: parotid gland.
C: submandibular gland.
D: gall bladder.
E: tongue.

Learning Response C: Correct. Mucous secretory cells are capped by serous secreting cells forming a serous demilune. These structures would be found in either the submandibular or sublingual gland. The tongue, pancreas and parotid gland do not have mucus secreting acinar cells.

438. SUBJECT AREA: Male Reproductive System

QUESTION: The blood-testis barrier is formed by

A: peritubular capillary endothelium.
B: Sertoli cells.
C: spermatocyte epithelium.
D: the basement membrane of the seminiferous tubule.
E: myoid cells.

Learning Response B: Correct. Protection from blood-borne products is the result of occluding junctions between Sertoli cells.

439. SUBJECT AREA: Male Reproductive System
QUESTION: Interstitial (Leydig) cell functions are controlled by

A: the pituitary gland.
B: the prostate.
C: secretions of the spermatids.
D: the number of spermatozoa.
E: smooth muscle contractions.

Learning Response A: Correct. Luteinizing hormone from the hypophysis stimulates testosterone synthesis by the interstitial (Leydig) cells.

440. SUBJECT AREA: Male Reproductive System
QUESTION: The convoluted regions of the seminiferous tubules of the testes empty directly into

A: the rete testis.
B: ductuli efferentes.
C: the epididymis.
D: the tubuli recti.
E: the seminal vesicles.

Learning Response D: Correct. The tubuli recti or straight tubules drain the seminiferous tubules and empty into the rete testis located in the mediastinum, a thickening of the tunica albuginea. From the rete testis the spermatozoa pass to the ductuli efferentes and from there to the epididymis.

441. SUBJECT AREA: Male Reproductive System
QUESTION: The epididymis

A: is lined by stratified columnar epithelium.
B: functions in the capacitation of sperm.
C: lacks smooth muscle fibers.
D: is lined by ciliated epithelium.
E: lacks blood vessels.

Learning Response B: Correct. The epididymis is a highly coiled tube extending from the efferent ductules to the vas deferens and is lined with pseudostratified epithelium. Its function is the capacitation of spermatozoa which enables them to attain a directed movement and renders them capable of fertilization.

---

442. SUBJECT AREA: Male Reproductive System

QUESTION: Spermatogonia have all of the following characteristics EXCEPT that they are

A: diploid cells.
B: susceptible to damage by body temperature.
C: present in both adult and fetal males.
D: capable of both mitosis and meiosis.
E: found closest to the lumen of the seminiferous tubules.

Learning Response E: Correct. The spermatogonia rest on the basal lamina of the seminiferous tubules and are farthest from the lumen.

---

443. SUBJECT AREA: Male Reproductive System

QUESTION: The testes are surrounded by a thick connective tissue capsule called the

A: tunica propria.
B: tunica albuginea.
C: tunica vaginalis.
D: tunica adventitia.
E: tunica dartos.

Learning Response B: Correct. The thick collagenous connective tissue that surrounds the testes is the tunica albuginea. The tunica vaginalis is a serous sac derived from peritoneal tissue and covers the tunica albuginea on the anterior and lateral sides of the testes. The tunica propria is the thin connective tissue that is adjacent to each seminiferous tubule.

444. SUBJECT AREA: Male Reproductive System
QUESTION: The interstitial cells of Leydig

A: become functional during the first two weeks of the neonatal period.
B: are located within the seminiferous tubule.
C: secrete much of the fluid portion of semen.
D: are stimulated by luteinizing hormone.
E: are enclosed by the layer of myoid cells.

Learning Response D: Correct. The interstitial cells are located in the interstitial connective tissue between the seminiferous tubules and are stimulated by luteinizing hormone from the anterior pituitary. They become functional at puberty. The majority of the fluid of semen is produced by the seminal vesicles. Myoid cells adhere to the basal lamina of the seminiferous tubules.

445. SUBJECT AREA: Male Reproductive System
QUESTION: Sertoli cells

A: produce androgen-binding protein to elevate the concentration of testosterone in the seminal vesicles.
B: synthesize and secrete inhibin which controls the secretion of pituitary luteinizing hormone.
C: together with the spermatogonia constitute the blood-testis barrier.
D: can be considered to be neuronal cells within the seminiferous tubules.
E: are phagocytic for cytoplasm removed from spermatids during spermiogenesis.

Learning Response E: Correct. During spermiogenesis, Sertoli cells remove the shed cytoplasm of the spermatids. Androgen-binding protein functions in the seminiferous tubules, not the seminal vesicles. Occluding junctions between Sertoli cells themselves form the blood-testis barrier. Inhibin is secreted by Sertoli cells, but the hormone functions to suppress pituitary FSH synthesis and release.

446. SUBJECT AREA: Male Reproductive System
QUESTION: In the production of male germ cells,

A: fully differentiated, motile spermatozoa are
released into the lumen of the seminiferous tubules.
B: each secondary spermatocyte, which is tetraploid,
undergoes meiotic division to form four haploid
cells.
C: after puberty the secretions of the anterior pituitary
have no effect on spermatogenesis.
D: type A spermatogonia give rise to primary
spermatocytes.
E: the acrosomal vesicle develops in the region of a
spermatid embedded in the Sertoli cell.

Learning Response E: Correct. The entire process of spermiogenesis occurs
while the spermatid is enclosed by the Sertoli cell. Type A spermatogonia are
undifferentiated stem cells whereas type B spermatogonia give rise to primary
spermatocytes. Secondary spermatocytes are haploid cells. Spermatozoa
released from the seminiferous tubules are not fully mature and cannot
undergo directed movements.

447. SUBJECT AREA: Male Reproductive System
QUESTION: The prostate gland

A: secretes citric acid, prostaglandins and acid
phosphatase.
B: has an anterior lobe which is most often associated
with the development of carcinomas.
C: functions primarily in the production of mucus
which clears the urethra and neutralizes any
residual urine present there.
D: secretes fructose which serves as the energy source
for sperm motility.
E: can exhibit calcified concretions which decrease in
number with advancing age of the individual.

Learning Response A: Correct. Prostatic carcinomas are most likely to be found in the posterior lobe. The numbers of prostatic concretions increase with age. The bulbourethral glands (also the glands of Littré) and seminal vesicles perform the functions described in choices C and D, respectively.

---

448. SUBJECT AREA: Male Reproductive System
QUESTION: Spermatids have all of the following features EXCEPT that they

A: are products of the second meiotic division of secondary spermatocytes.
B: are located next to the lumen of the seminiferous tubules.
C: may exhibit an acrosome which contains several hydrolytic enzymes.
D: are capable of mitosis.
E: may exhibit a cylinder of microtubules, the manchette, which surrounds the nucleus.

Learning Response D: Correct. Spermatids are the result of the division of secondary spermatocytes and are postmitotic.

---

449. SUBJECT AREA: Male Reproductive System
QUESTION: The seminiferous tubules

A: include a myoid cell layer located most peripherally.
B: contain testosterone secreting cells.
C: contain Sertoli cells which rest on the basal lamina.
D: exhibit only features in A and C above.
E: exhibit features in A, B and C above.

Learning Response D: Correct. Myoid cells are the outermost cells of the seminiferous tubules, and they and the Sertoli cells are associated with the basal lamina. Testosterone secreting cells are located in the interstitial connective tissue between the seminiferous tubules.

450. SUBJECT AREA: Male Reproductive System
QUESTION: In the male reproductive system,

A: temperature is unimportant for the development of spermatozoa.
B: the seminal vesicles secrete an abundance of glucose to provide energy for sperm movements.
C: prostatic concretions are crystals of magnesium sulfate.
D: the penile corpora cavernosae are surrounded by dense connective tissue.
E: both the seminal vesicles and the prostate lack smooth muscle fibers.

Learning Response D: Correct. The erectile tissue of the corpora cavernosae in the penis is surrounded by a thick band of connective tissue called the tunica albuginea. The seminal vesicles secrete fructose as the primary carbohydrate energy source for sperm. Temperature plays a role in spermatogenesis with normal testicular temperature about 2° C lower than normal body temperature. Prostatic concretions are often calcified.

451 SUBJECT AREA: Male Reproductive System
QUESTION: Sperm pass through all of the following EXCEPT

A: the tubuli recti which are lined by cuboidal epithelial tissue.
B: the ductus deferens which contains smooth muscle layers.
C: the epididymis which is lined by pseudostratified columnar epithelium.
D: the ductuli which lead to the epididymis.
E: the rete testis which is a straight tubule penetrating the mediastinum.

Learning Response E: Correct. The seminiferous tubules empty into the tubuli recti or straight tubules. The tubuli recti lead to the rete testis, an anastomosing network of channels which traverse the mediastinum testis. From there the spermatozoa enter the efferent ductules which fuse to form the epididymis in which sperm acquire their ability to fertilize ova.

---

452. SUBJECT AREA: Male Reproductive System
QUESTION: The peritoneal layer that covers the anterior and lateral aspects of the testis is known as the

A: tunica propria.
B: tunica vaginalis.
C: tunica albuginea.
D: tunica dartos.
E: tunica adventitia.

Learning Response B: Correct. The outer parietal and inner visceral layers of the tunica vaginalis cover the testis and are derived from the peritoneum during the descent of the testis into the scrotal sac.

---

453. SUBJECT AREA: Male Reproductive System
QUESTION: Primary spermatocytes are

A: haploid.
B: diploid.
C: tetraploid.
D: postmitotic.
E: 2N in the amount of DNA.

Learning Response B: Correct. The amount of DNA in primary spermatocytes is 4N, and they are diploid cells with 2N (46) in chromosome number.

---

454. SUBJECT AREA: Male Reproductive System
QUESTION: All of the following occur during spermiogenesis EXCEPT

A: the accumulation of PAS positive granules in the Golgi complex of spermatids.
B: elongation of spermatid nucleus.
C: the reorganization of mitochondria along the

proximal portion of the flagellum.

D: activation of acrosomal lysosomal enzymes that hydrolyze the intercellular bridges between spermatids.

E: microtubules extend from one of the centrioles of the spermatid to form the flagellum.

Learning Response D: Correct. When spermatozoa encounter an ovum, the outer acrosome membrane fuses with the plasmalemma of the sperm cells. The acrosomal lysosomal enzymes are liberated and begin digesting the zona pellucida and corona radiata of the ovum.

---

455. SUBJECT AREA: Male Reproductive System
QUESTION: Identify the structure depicted in the figure below.

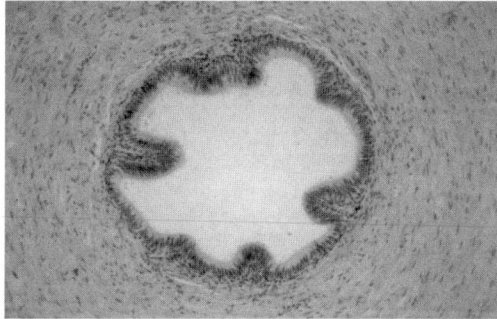

A: epididymis
B: ductus (vas) deferens
C: efferent ductule
D: seminal vesicle
E: straight tubule

Learning Response B: Correct. The historical characteristics of the ductus deferens include a narrow lumen lined by pseudostratified epithelium which has stereocillia, a lamina propria rich in elastic fibers and a thick coat of smooth muscle arranged in three distinct layers.

456. SUBJECT AREA: Male Reproductive System
QUESTION: A defect in the gene coding for follicle stimulating hormone (FSH) would probably result in

A: a decrease in the amount of androgen-binding protein secreted by Sertoli cells.
B: a reduction in the amounts of testosterone transported to the seminiferous tubules.
C: a reduction in the amounts of inhibin secreted by Sertoli cells.
D: a reduction in the numbers of spermatozoa.
E: all of the above effects.

Learning Response E: Correct. Most likely all of the events listed would be affected by defects in FSH which, among other functions, stimulates the synthesis of androgen-binding protein.

457. SUBJECT AREA: Male Reproductive System
QUESTION: The primary function of the blood-testis barrier is

A: the protection of the spermatogenic cells from an autoimmune reaction.
B: to allow select immunoglobulins into the seminiferous epithelium to protect it from microorganisms.
C: the protection of germ cells from neutrophils in the interstitial tissue of the seminiferous tubules.
D: to permit a one way migration of germ cells from basal lamina to lumen of the seminiferous tubules.
E: to prevent the movement of Leydig cells into the seminiferous tubules.

Learning Response A: Correct. Since the onset of sexual maturity takes place well after the development of the immune system, the differentiating sperm cells might be recognized as foreign and thus stimulate an immune response against them. The blood-testis barrier effectively eliminates any interaction between the developing germ cells and the immune system.

458. SUBJECT AREA: Male Reproductive System
QUESTION: All of the following are features of the prostate EXCEPT

A: the separation of the gland into lobes by connective tissue septa.
B: that it is composed of two distinct groups of glandular epithelia.
C: an abundance of smooth muscle fibers surrounds the epithelium.
D: the secretion of most of the seminal fluid in the ejaculate.
E: the presence of concentrated bodies of glycoprotein in the glandular lumen.

Learning Response D: Correct. The seminal vesicle secretes 70% of the fluid in the ejaculate.

459. SUBJECT AREA: Male Reproductive System
QUESTION: The interstitial cells of Leydig would have all of the following organelles and inclusions EXCEPT

A: stacks of rough endoplasmic reticulum.
B: an abundance of smooth endoplasmic reticulum.
C: a rich supply of lipid droplets.
D: mitochondria to provide the energy for hormone synthesis.
E: centrally located nuclei.

Learning Response A: Correct. The interstitial cells are typical steroid-secreting cells and have the organelles and inclusions to reflect that activity.

460. SUBJECT AREA: Male Reproductive System
QUESTION: All of the following cells are adluminal in relation to the basal lamina of the seminiferous tubules EXCEPT

A: spermatids.
B: spermatogonia.
C: myoid cells.
D: Sertoli cells.
E: secondary spermatocytes.

Learning Response C: Correct. The myoid cells rest on the basal lamina adjacent to the interstitial tissue On the opposite side of the basal lamina reside the germinal cells and the Sertoli cells.

461. SUBJECT AREA: Male Reproductive System
QUESTION: The bulbourethral glands (Cowper's glands)

A: are simple tubular glands.
B: are located distal to the membranous portion of the urethra.
C: are lined by simple squamous epithelium.
D: secrete fructose, citrate and inositol for the activation of sperm.
E: have both smooth and skeletal muscle in septa which divide the glands into lobes.

Learning Response E: Correct. The tubuloalveolar bulbourethral glands are proximal to the membranous urethra and are lined with mucus secreting simple cuboidal epithelium.

462. SUBJECT AREA: Male Reproductive System
QUESTION: The major clinical significance of the submucosal and main glands of the prostate is that

A: their hyperplasia is the source of benign prostatic hypertrophy.
B: their location accounts for their susceptibility to bacterial infection.
C: they can be the source of malignant cells causing cancer of the prostate.
D: their proximity to blood vessels can lead to autoimmune reactions against the gland cells.

E: their malfunction can lead to immotile spermatozoa syndrome.

Learning Response C: Correct. Prostatic carcinoma is the second most common form of cancer in males and the third leading cause of cancer related deaths.

463. SUBJECT AREA: Female Reproductive System

QUESTION: Each of the following statements pertaining to the oogonia (primary germ cells) is true EXCEPT

A: the oogonia cannot be identified in the endodermal yolk sac prior to the first month of embryonic life.

B: mitotic division occurs several times during the migration of the oogonia to the genital ridge.

C: they populate the medulla of the ovary.

D: mitotic division continues to about the fifth month of fetal life, giving rise to more than 3 million oogonia.

E: they enter prophase of the first meiotic division by the end of the seventh month of fetal life.

Learning Response C: Correct. Oogonia reside in the cortex of the ovary.

464. SUBJECT AREA: Female Reproductive System

QUESTION: The following structures are characteristic of a primary follicle EXCEPT

A: layers of granulosa cells.

B: antrum.

C: theca interna.

D: basal lamina.

E: zona pellucida.

Learning Response B: Correct. The antrum contains an accumulation of follicular fluid. The formation of an antrum is coincident with the commencement of the secondary follicle stage of development.

465. SUBJECT AREA: Female Reproductive System
QUESTION: Follicle atresia

A: results from the degradation of granulosa cells thus causing the death of the oocyte.
B: occurs only after birth.
C: is greatest at menopause.
D: only occurs in secondary follicles.
E: is caused by a lack of O_2 from the blood supply.

Learning Response A: Correct. Granulosa cells and oocytes have a paracrine relationship. The oocytes contain receptors for a substance known as SCF (stem cell factor) which is synthesized and secreted by the granulosa cells. SCF promotes the survival of the oocytes and prevents apoptosis (programmed cell death) from occurring.

466. SUBJECT AREA: Female Reproductive System
QUESTION: Ovarian androgens are produced by the

A: pituitary.
B: theca externa cells.
C: zona pellucida.
D: interstitial cells.
E: granulosa cells.

Learning Response D: Correct. Interstitial cells are active steroid secreting thecal cells. They are present from childhood through menopause and are the main source of ovarian androgens.

467. SUBJECT AREA: Female Reproductive System
QUESTION: Ovulation

A: occurs approximately on the 21st day of a 28 day menstrual cycle.
B: is accompanied by a surge of luteinizing hormone (LH) concentration.
C: results in the disappearance of the germinal epithelium.

>   *D:* releases the ovum together with the follicular
>   liquid, granulosa cells and the theca interna.
>   *E:* is initiated by contractions of the ovarian smooth
>   muscle cells which push the mature follicle toward
>   the surface of the ovary.

Learning Response B: Correct. LH is synthesized by the pars distalis of the pituitary. It stimulates the granulosa and the theca interna cells of the ruptured follicle to become steroid secreting lutein cells of the corpus luteum. Ovulation usually occurs at approximately the midpoint of the cycle.

---

468. SUBJECT AREA: Female Reproductive System
>   QUESTION: Each of the following statements with respect to the
>   corpus luteum is true EXCEPT that it

>   *A:* is an exocrine gland.
>   *B:* secretes progesterone which prevents the
>   development of new follicles and the occurrence of
>   ovulation.
>   *C:* consists of 80% steroid secreting granulosa lutein
>   cells that were once the protein secreting granulosa
>   cells.
>   *D:* produces progesterone which inhibits the
>   production of luteinizing hormone.
>   *E:* is maintained for six months in the presence of
>   chorionic gonadotropin produced by the placenta.

Learning Response A: Correct. The corpus luteum functions as an endocrine gland and secretes its products into the interstitial space where they diffuse to capillaries.

---

469. SUBJECT AREA: Female Reproductive System
>   QUESTION: Relaxin

>   *A:* softens the connective tissue of the symphysis
>   pubis facilitating parturition.
>   *B:* is secreted by the hypothalamus.
>   *C:* is secreted by the corpus albicans.

D: relaxes the abdominal muscles during parturition.
E: has none of the above characteristics.

Learning Response A: Correct. Relaxin is a polypeptide secreted by the corpus luteum. It softens the connective tissue of the symphysis pubis during parturition.

---

470. SUBJECT AREA: Female Reproductive System
QUESTION: The wall of the oviduct

A: is lined with simple columnar cells with stereocilia.
B: is composed of three layers: mucosa, muscularis and an external adventitia.
C: is most highly folded throughout the intramural portion.
D: contains cells with cilia and cells that are secretory.
E: has cells that secrete a viscous substance which protects the epithelial lining.

Learning Response D: Correct. Two types of cells line the lumenal wall of the oviduct. One cell type has cilia that beat mainly toward the uterus moving the viscous liquid toward that direction. Some cilia beat in the opposite direction (toward the ovary) and may facilitate the movement of the sperm toward the ovum. The second cell type is secretory and has short microvilli. It secretes a viscous liquid which nourishes and protects the ovum as well as moves it toward the uterus. The secretory cells also promote the activation of spermatozoa. The oviduct is covered with peritoneum, and hence, has an outer layer of serosa, not adventitia.

---

471. SUBJECT AREA: Female Reproductive System
QUESTION: All of the following can occur in the oviduct at ovulation EXCEPT

A: the lumen of the oviduct maintains an environment sufficient for fertilization.
B: infundibular fimbriae move closer to the surface of the ovary to facilitate capture of the ovum.
C: the blood vessels of the oviduct become dilated.

D: fertilization normally occurs in the first half of the oviduct.

E: the lamina propria of the oviduct can react like the endometrium if the fertilized ovum implants itself in the wall of the oviduct.

Learning Response D: Correct. Fertilization usually takes place in the lateral third of the oviduct.

472. SUBJECT AREA: Female Reproductive System
QUESTION The uterus

A: is the only place implantation of a fertilized egg can occur.

B: physiologically changes only during pregnancy.

C: is lined with simple columnar epithelium that contains cells that are either ciliated or secretory.

D: undergoes cyclic changes which are initiated by progesterone.

E: contains a myometrium which consists of a functional zone and a basal zone.

Learning Response C: Correct. The surface epithelium of the endometrium consists of ciliated and secretory cells. Ciliated cells are rarely seen within the uterine glands.

473. SUBJECT AREA: Female Reproductive System
QUESTION: During pregnancy,

A: the endometrium sloughs off its functional layer.

B: the increase in progesterone levels causes the cervical glands to secrete a fluid and highly nutritious substance for the fertilized egg.

C: the growth of the myometrium is due to hypertrophy, not hyperplasia.

D: smooth muscle cells of the myometrium actively synthesize collagen.

E: all of the above events can occur.

Learning Response D: Correct. Pregnancy causes the smooth muscle cells in the myometrium to synthesize collagen actively, thus significantly increasing the uterine collagen content. Following pregnancy, the enzymatic degradation of the collagen aids in the reduction in size of the uterus.

---

474. SUBJECT AREA: Female Reproductive System
QUESTION: Cervical secretions

> A: play an insignificant role in the fertilization of the ovum.
> B: are highly viscous at the time of ovulation in order to prevent microorganisms from infecting the ovum.
> C: only occur at parturition.
> D: can form nabothian cysts when cervical glands become blocked.
> E: are characterized by none of the above choices.

Learning Response D: Correct. Cervical glands located near the external os are most likely to become blocked. The mucin produced within these glands accumulates and produces spherical cystic masses of mucus lined by a flattened, endocervical mucus secreting epithelium.

---

475. SUBJECT AREA: Female Reproductive System
QUESTION: Carcinoma of the cervix

> A: is most commonly found at the transformation zone of the cervical stratified squamous epithelium.
> B: cannot be detected until it is in the later stages.
> C: has a high mortality rate.
> D: has cells that have a regular stratified appearance with a low nucleus-to-cytoplasmic ratio.
> E: can be treated with sulfur drugs.

Learning Response A: Correct. Cervical cancer is usually detected at or near the transformation zone of the cervical epithelium. Early diagnosis is obtained by cervical smear (cells are scraped from the epithelial surface in the region of the external os). Abnormal areas can usually be treated by surgical removal with a low mortality rate (8 per 100,000).

476. SUBJECT AREA: Female Reproductive System
   QUESTION: The proliferative phase of the menstrual cycle

> *A:* begins on the 7th day and ends of the 14th day of the cycle.
> *B:* is characterized by the presence of uterine glands that are highly coiled.
> *C:* is initiated by the secretion of estrogen from the granulosa cells of the maturing follicle in the ovary.
> *D:* is initiated by the secretion of progesterone from the follicle theca interna cells in the ovary.
> *E:* is also known as the luteal phase.

Learning Response C: Correct. The proliferative phase, also known as the follicular phase, is initiated when estrogen secretion from the granulosa cells of the maturing follicle commences. As the estrogen level increases, so does the height of the endometrium. The presence of coiled uterine glands is a feature of the secretory stage of the cycle.

477. SUBJECT AREA: Female Reproductive System
   QUESTION: During the secretory phase of the menstrual cycle,

> *A:* the endometrium reaches its maximum thickness.
> *B:* the epithelial cells of the glands of the uterus begin to accumulate glycogen.
> *C:* glycoprotein secretory products empty into the lumen of the glands.
> *D:* glands become tortuous and their lumen becomes dilated.
> *E:* all of the above events occur.

Learning Response E: Correct. The secretory phase begins after ovulation and lasts from about day 6 to day 25. This phase occurs in response to progesterone secretion by the corpus luteum. Progesterone stimulates the uterine glands to secrete glycoproteins.

478. SUBJECT AREA: Female Reproductive System
QUESTION: In the event of a successful fertilization and implantation,

   A: progesterone secreted from the corpus luteum immediately stops.
   B: the embryo is totally embedded in the endometrium at the 9th to the 11th day after ovulation.
   C: the latter takes place when the endometrium is in the proliferative stage.
   D: the fertilized cell mass is known as a morula at the time of implantation.
   E: uterine arteries are reduced in height to postmenstrual levels.

Learning Response B: Correct. The endometrium is in the secretory phase at the time the blastocyst gains access to the endometrial stroma. This occurs approximately 9 to 11 days after ovulation.

479. SUBJECT AREA: Female Reproductive System
QUESTION: The developing zygote

   A: undergoes a series of mitotic divisions, immediately after fertilization, to produce a solid ball of cells known as a morula.
   B: enters the endometrial cavity before it divides into the morula stage.
   C: will degenerate if it does not successfully implant itself in the endometrium.
   D: implants itself in the endometrium as soon as it enters the uterus.
   E: when at the blastocyst stage, has a solid collection of cells at one pole, known as the inner cell mass, which will give rise to the umbilical cord.

Learning Response A: Correct. The ovum becomes fertilized at the ampulla-isthmus junction of the oviduct. Cleavage of the zygote occurs. As the fertilized ovum moves down the oviduct, it undergoes a series of mitotic divisions until it forms a compact collection of cells called a morula.

480. SUBJECT AREA: Female Reproductive System
QUESTION: Syncytiotrophoblast cells

A: are mononucleated, ovoid cells surrounding the
cytotrophoblast.
B: secrete chorionic gonadotropin, placental lactogen,
estrogen and progesterone.
C: secrete growth hormone.
D: have an abundance of rough endoplasmic
reticulum, indicative of a protein secreting cell.
E: have all of the above features.

Learning Response B: Correct. Syncytiotrophoblast cells contain a large
amount of both rough and smooth endoplasmic reticulum, a well developed
Golgi complex, lipid droplets and an abundance of mitochondria. These
organelles are associated with both peptide and steroid hormonal secretion.
The syncytiotrophoblast cells synthesize chorionic gonadotropin, placental
lactogen, estrogen and progesterone.

481. SUBJECT AREA: Female Reproductive System
QUESTION: Decidua basalis cells of the endometrium are

A: found between the embryo and the lumen of the
uterus.
B: found between the embryo and the myometrium.
C: found throughout the entire endometrium.
D: continually renewing cytotrophoblast cells.
E: found in the endometrium prior to implantation of
the fertilized ovum.

Learning Response B: Correct. Decidua basalis cells of the endometrium are
found between the embryo and the myometrium. These cells are large in size
and exhibit features of protein synthesizing cells producing, among other
substances, prolactin.

482. SUBJECT AREA: Female Reproductive System
QUESTION: The placenta

A: is formed by the decidua basalis of the endometrium.

B: takes the place of the endometrium.

C: is the only organ composed of cells derived from two different individuals.

D: is maintained by glucocorticoids secreted by the zona fasciculata of the adrenal.

E: has tertiary villi which contain maternal blood.

Learning Response C: Correct. The placenta is a temporary organ consisting of a fetal portion, formed by the chorion, and a maternal portion, formed by the decidua basalis. The placenta is the site of physiological exchanges between the mother and the fetal circulation.

---

483. SUBJECT AREA: Female Reproductive System
QUESTION: The mucosa of the vagina

A: is normally lined by stratified columnar cells.

B: is normally lined by keratinized stratified squamous epithelium.

C: lacks elastic fibers.

D: secretes progesterone.

E: stores glycogen.

Learning Response E: Correct. The vaginal wall is composed of three layers: mucosa, muscularis and adventitia. The epithelial lining consists of nonkeratinized stratified squamous cells which synthesize and accumulate large quantities of glycogen after stimulation by estrogen. The lamina propria under the epithelium is rich in elastic fibers. There are no glands in the vaginal wall.

---

484. SUBJECT AREA: Female Reproductive System
QUESTION: The endometrium

A: may contain only one layer known as the functionalis.

B: lies internal to the myometrium and is composed of smooth muscle.

C: responds to mineralocorticoids by forming
extended endometrial glands.

D: secretes testosterone.

E: has a vascular supply associated with the
functionalis that is destroyed with each cycle.

Learning Response E: Correct. The endometrium contains two sets of arteries
which arise from the arcuate arteries originating in the middle layers of the
myometrium. These arteries are: straight arteries, which supply the basalis
and coiled arteries, which supply the functionalis.

485. SUBJECT AREA: Female Reproductive System
QUESTION: The mammary gland

A: is a simple alveolar structure.

B: secretes its milk through ducts by the action of
myoepithelial cells which encircle the ductal cells.

C: has myoepithelial cells which contract when
exposed to prolactin.

D: has secretory alveoli which will remain intact when
milk is not removed.

E: has ducts which grow in response to luteal
progesterone.

Learning Response B: Correct. Oxytocin elicits contraction of myoepithelial
cells in alveoli and ducts of the mammary gland causing a milk-ejection
reflex.

486. SUBJECT AREA: Female Reproductive System
QUESTION: The oocyte in a secondary follicle is separated from the
follicular cells of the cumulus oophorus by the

A: theca interna.

B: zona glomerulosa.

C: zona pellucida.

D: zona fasciculata.

E: theca externa.

Learning Response C: Correct. The zona pellucida is a distinct glycoprotein layer of eosinophilic (PAS-positive) material which forms between the oocyte and the granulosa cells.

---

487. SUBJECT AREA: Female Reproductive System
QUESTION: If pregnancy does not occur, the corpus luteum begins to degenerate and ultimately becomes a(n)

   A: corpus hemorrhagicum.
   B: corpus albicans.
   C: Graafian follicle.
   D: primordial follicle.
   E: atretic follicle.

Learning Response B: Correct. The cells of the corpus luteum undergo degeneration by autolysis. What remains behind is a scar of dense connective tissue known as a corpus albicans which remains for a variable period of time before it is absorbed by phagocytic cells in the ovarian stroma.

---

488. SUBJECT AREA: Female Reproductive System
QUESTION: The mammary gland

   A: evidences lobuloalveolar growth in response to ovarian hormones with the onset of puberty.
   B: exhibits no cyclical changes with each menstrual cycle.
   C: secretes lipids and proteins by similar mechanisms.
   D: is aided in emptying its contents by neurosecretory impulses that release oxytocin from the posterior pituitary.
   E: has neuromuscular junctions that function to express milk from the alveoli.

Learning Response D: Correct. The nursing action of the infant stimulates tactile receptors in the nipple which results in the release of oxytocin from the posterior pituitary. Oxytocin causes the myoepithelial cells to contract in the alveoli and ducts, resulting in the release of milk.

489. SUBJECT AREA: Female Reproductive System
QUESTION: All of the following statements about the placenta are true EXCEPT that it

A: secretes hormones which support the function of the corpus luteum.
B: provides no barrier to transmission of viruses such as rubella, smallpox or measles to the embryo.
C: has increased numbers of cytotrophoblast cells as pregnancy progresses.
D: modifies its functions to accommodate the development of the embryo.
E: can, during some pregnancies, pass fetal red blood cells into the maternal circulation initiating a condition known as erythroblastosis fetalis.

Learning Response C: Correct. The number of cytotrophoblast cells decreases as pregnancy progresses.

490. SUBJECT AREA: Female Reproductive System
QUESTION: In reference to the mammary gland,

A: lactation depends on the presence of a functional adrenal cortex.
B: vasoconstriction caused by epinephrine release can inhibit lactation by blocking the effects of oxytocin.
C: IgA may be transferred from the mother to the child in milk.
D: parathyroid hormone assists in the maintenance of calcium levels in its secretions.
E: all of the above statements are correct.

Learning Response E: Correct. The mammary gland exhibits all of the features listed above.

491. SUBJECT AREA: Female Reproductive System
QUESTION: Which phase of the uterine menstrual cycle is depicted in the figure below?

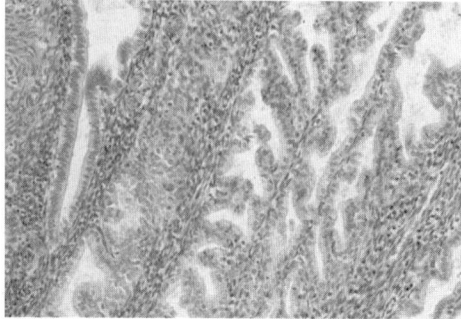

A: proliferative phase
B: resting phase
C: early menstruation phase
D: secretory phase
E: late menstruation phase

Learning Response D: Correct. The lumen of the uterine glands becomes highly coiled and the epithelial cells are dilated by the accumulation of secretory material.

492. SUBJECT AREA: Female Reproductive System
QUESTION: Identify the layer of cells lying just beneath the outer layer of the chorionic villi shown in the figure below.

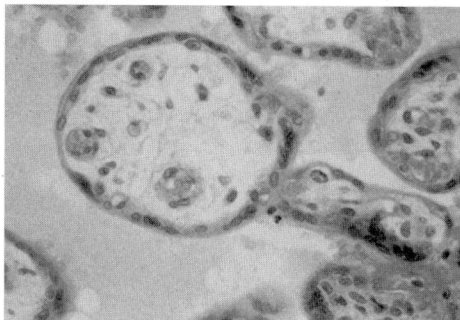

> *A:* syncytiotrophoblast
> *B:* cytotrophoblast
> *C:* basal lamina
> *D:* decidua basalis
> *E:* mesenchyme

Learning Response B: Correct. Cytotrophoblast cells form a discontinuous layer of cells just beneath the syncytiotrophoblast. Their nuclei are larger and stain lighter than those of syncytiotrophoblastic cells.

---

493. SUBJECT AREA: Female Reproductive System
QUESTION: The labia minora of the female external genitalia

> *A:* have very few sensory tactile nerve endings.
> *B:* are formed by two erectile bodies.
> *C:* consist of the clitoris and the labia majora.
> *D:* contain sebaceous and sweat glands on the inner and outer surfaces.
> *E:* have an abundance of adipose tissue.

Learning Response D: Correct. The labia minora are folds of skin with a central core of connective tissue containing elastic fibers. Sebaceous and sweat glands are located just beneath the inner and outer surfaces of stratified squamous epithelium. The clitoris is formed by two erectile bodies and the labia majora contain large quantities of adipose tissue.

---

494. SUBJECT AREA: Female Reproductive System
QUESTION: Which cells of the corpus luteum are derived from the ovarian stroma?

> *A:* theca lutein cells
> *B:* granulosa lutein cells
> *C:* follicular cells
> *D:* germinal epithelium
> *E:* corona radiata cells

Learning Response A: Correct. After ovulation the cells of the theca interna become the theca lutein cells and contribute to the function of the corpus luteum.

---

495. SUBJECT AREA: Female Reproductive System
QUESTION: The myometrium

> *A:* increases in mass during pregnancy by hyperplasia.
> *B:* increases in mass during pregnancy by hypertrophy.
> *C:* contracts in response to oxytocin.
> *D:* remains intact during menstruation.
> *E:* can exhibit all of the above features.

Learning Response E: Correct. It should be emphasized that growth of the uterus during pregnancy occurs by both hypertrophy and hyperplasia. All of the above responses are characteristic of the myometrium.

---

496. SUBJECT AREA: Female Reproductive System
QUESTION: Colostrum

> *A:* contains primarily lipids.
> *B:* is released immediately following birth.
> *C:* is an incomplete form of milk produced by hormonally deficient mothers.
> *D:* contains antibodies produced by plasma cells in the mammary interlobular connective tissue.
> *E:* is characterized by choices B and D above.

Learning Response E: Correct. Colostrum, which is rich in proteins, conveys passive immunity to the child through its content of immunoglobulin A (IgA). Although colostrum is the first secretion of the breast after the birth of the child, its release usually begins approximately two days postpartum.

---

497. SUBJECT AREA: Female Reproductive System
QUESTION: Identify the structure depicted in the figure below.

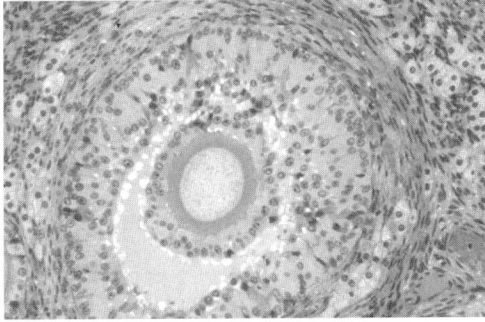

A: atretic follicle
B: primordial follicle
C: primary follicle
D: secondary follicle
E: Graafian follicle

Learning Response D: Correct. The presence of an antrum which separates the outer granulosa cells from the corona radiata cells surrounding the oocyte is the major clue in the identification of this structure. The antrum houses accumulations of follicular liquid containing transudates of plasma and products secreted by the follicular cells such as steroids and glycosaminoglycans.

498. SUBJECT AREA: Urinary System
QUESTION: Renin can be located in the cells of the

        A: macula densa.
        B: proximal convoluted tubule.
        C: distal convoluted tubule.
        D: afferent arteriole.
        E: efferent arteriole.

Learning Response D: Correct. Smooth muscle cells in the tunica media of the afferent arteriole synthesize and secrete the hormone renin which acts to elevate blood pressure. These cells are known as juxtaglomerular cells.

499. SUBJECT AREA: Urinary System

QUESTION: In the medulla of the kidney, the collecting tubules coalesce to form structures called

A: area cribosa.
B: medullary rays.
C: thick loops of Henle.
D: papillary ducts.
E: renal calyces.

Learning Response D: Correct. Papillary ducts, which lead into the area cribosa at the apex of the renal pyramid, are lined with simple columnar epithelium and are formed by the union of collecting ducts which are lined by simple cuboidal epithelium. Medullary rays are cortical structures which contain elements of the tubules leading from cortex to medulla and vice versa.

500. SUBJECT AREA: Urinary System
QUESTION: The proximal tubules of the kidney

A: are composed of simple squamous epithelium.
B: exhibit numerous microvilli at the cell surface.
C: secrete glucose and amino acids into the glomerular filtrate.
D: lack a basal lamina.
E: are continuous with collecting ducts.

Learning Response B: Correct. The simple cuboidal epithelial cells of the proximal tubules function to reabsorb glucose and amino acids from the glomerular filtrate The presence of microvilli as a brush border on their apical surface increases the absorptive area. As epithelial cells, they rest on a basal lamina. The proximal tubules are drained by the thin segment of Henle's loop.

501. SUBJECT AREA: Urinary System
QUESTION: The cells of the visceral layer of renal corpuscle are called

A: mesangial cells.
B: podocytes.

> C: juxtaglomerular cells.
> D: macula densa cells.
> E: extraglomerular mesangial cells.

Learning Response B: Correct. Podocytes are specialized cells of the visceral layer of the renal corpuscle. They rest on the glomerular basement membrane and contribute to the process of glomerular filtration. Intraglomerular mesangial cells are located in the connective tissue between the capillary loops of the glomerulus. Juxtaglomerular cells are found in the walls of the afferent arterioles. Macula densa cells are part of the distal tubule which is extraglomerular.

502. SUBJECT AREA: Urinary System
QUESTION: The distal convoluted tubules (dct) of the kidney

> A: are composed of simple cuboidal epithelium.
> B: have a well developed brush border.
> C: secrete glucose and amino acids into the glomerular filtrate.
> D: lack a basement membrane.
> E: have numerous ribosomes associated with basal membrane invaginations.

Learning Response A: Correct. The distal convoluted tubules of the kidney are lined by simple cuboidal epithelium with a basement membrane, but not a brush border. The dct absorbs sodium and secretes potassium (in the presence of aldosterone), hydrogen and ammonium ions. Thus, the dct plays a key role in acid-base balance and contains many basal membrane invaginations with associated mitochondria to provide ATP to the ion pumps necessary to perform this function.

503. SUBJECT AREA: Urinary System
QUESTION: The juxtaglomerular (JG) apparatus is characterized by all of the following EXCEPT that it

> A: is located at the vascular pole of the renal corpuscle.
> B: includes mesangial cells located within the glomerulus.

C: includes cells that would be extremely active
following a significant hemorrhage.

D: includes cells of the macula densa.

E: includes cells found in a portion of the afferent
arteriole.

Learning Response B: Correct. The JG apparatus is composed of JG cells and the macula densa, a modified area of the distal tubule located at its point of contact with the vascular pole of the renal corpuscle. JG cells are modified smooth muscle cells found in the tunica media of the afferent arteriole. These cells secrete renin, an enzyme which ultimately leads to the formation of angiotensin II, a potent vasoconstrictor. As blood pressure falls following a significant hemorrhage, JG cells would be very active following such an event in an attempt to raise blood pressure. Intraglomerular mesangial cells are not included in this structure. However, extraglomerular mesangial cells (polkissen cells) are part of the JG apparatus.

504. SUBJECT AREA: Urinary System

QUESTION: Papillary ducts (also called collecting ducts)

A: exhibit distinct cell to cell boundaries.

B: are lined by simple columnar epithelium.

C: function in the urine-concentrating mechanism of
the kidney.

D: can respond to antidiuretic hormone (vasopressin).

E: can exhibit all of the above characteristics.

Learning Response E: Correct. Urine flows from the distal convoluted tubules to collecting tubules which are lined by simple cuboidal epithelium and then into collecting ducts, the epithelium of which is responsive to antidiuretic hormone. This hormone makes the epithelium of the collecting ducts permeable to water and allows for the formation of a concentrated, hypertonic urine.

505. SUBJECT AREA: Urinary System

QUESTION: Podocytes

A: contain secondary processes (pedicels) which are in

direct contact with the basal lamina.

B: contain secondary processes (pedicels) which may
be in contact with more than one capillary.

C: form the visceral layer of Bowman's capsule.

D: contain actin microfilaments.

E: are characterized by all of the above features.

Learning Response E: Correct. Podocytes, which form the visceral layer of
Bowman's capsule, have cell bodies and primary processes that do not rest on
the basal lamina. However, their secondary processes (pedicels) are in direct
contact with the basal lamina of the capillary at a regular distance of 25 nm.
In addition, the pedicels from one podocyte are in contact with more than one
capillary. On any given capillary, the pedicels of two different podocytes
alternate in a fashion which produces 25 nm-wide filtration slits. The
presence of actin microfilaments allows the pedicels to change their shape.

506. SUBJECT AREA: Urinary System
QUESTION: Which association is NOT correct?

A: proximal convoluted tubule—simple cuboidal or
columnar epithelium with brush border

B: urinary bladder—transitional epithelium

C: distal convoluted tubule—simple cuboidal
epithelium

D: ureter—columnar epithelium with brush border

E: interstitial cells—prostaglandin production

Learning Response D: Correct. The mucosa of the calyces, pelvis, ureter and
bladder have the same basic histological structure, and all of these structures
are lined with transitional epithelium.

507. SUBJECT AREA: Urinary System
QUESTION: The glomerular basement membrane

A: is derived from the fusion of capillary and
podocyte-produced basal laminae.

B: contains type IV collagen in the lamina rara which
acts as a physical filter for macromolecules.

C: contains heparan sulfate in the lamina densa which acts as a barrier to negatively charged particles.

D: is a privileged site that is not affected in disease states (e.g., diabetes mellitus).

E: is characterized by all of the above features.

Learning Response A: Correct. The glomerular basement membrane is derived from fusion of capillary and podocyte-produced basal lamina. The membrane is both a mechanical and electrical barrier: type IV collagen in the lamina densa and negatively charged heparan sulfate in the lamina rara restrict passage of particles greater than 10 nm in diameter or negatively charged proteins greater than 69,000 molecular weight. The glomerular basement membrane is often involved in disease processes, such as diabetes mellitus, where damage to the basement membrane results in increased permeability and subsequent proteinuria.

---

508. SUBJECT AREA: Urinary System

QUESTION: All of the following are true of juxtaglomerular cells EXCEPT

A: their secretions play a role in the maintenance of blood pressure.

B: their secretions ultimately lead to the formation of angiotensin II.

C: they are modified smooth muscle cells.

D: they contain rough endoplasmic reticulum, a highly developed Golgi complex and secretory granules.

E: they are found in a modified segment of the wall of the distal tubule.

Learning Response E: Correct. Juxtaglomerular cells are modified smooth muscle cells in the tunica media of the afferent arteriole that is in close proximity to the renal corpuscle. JG cells secrete the protein renin, and, therefore, have all the characteristics of protein-secreting cells described in choice D. Renin acts on a plasma protein, angiotensinogen, to produce angiotensin I, which is converted in the lung to angiontensin II, a potent vasoconstrictor that assists in the maintenance of blood pressure.

509. SUBJECT AREA: Urinary System
QUESTION: Mesangial cells

A: comprise the parietal layer of Bowman's capsule.
B: are restricted to the renal corpuscle.
C: secrete creatinine into the glomerular filtrate.
D: secrete proteins which contribute to the maintenance of blood pressure.
E: synthesize matrix proteins which help support the glomerular capillary walls.

Learning Response E: Correct. The parietal layer of Bowman's capsule consists of simple squamous epithelium. Intraglomerular mesangial cells are located in the interstitial tissue of the glomerulus between the capillary loops and may function in the maintenance of the glomerular basement membrane. Extraglomerular mesangial cells are located at the vascular pole of the renal corpuscle and are part of the JG apparatus; their function is uncertain. Secretion of creatinine into the glomerular filtrate is a function of the proximal convoluted tubule.

510. SUBJECT AREA: Urinary System
QUESTION: Endothelial cells of the glomerular capillaries are characterized by all of the following EXCEPT that they

A: form the lining of one side of the urinary space.
B: are fenestrated with numerous openings without diaphragms.
C: have unique modifications which enable them to participate in filtration.
D: rest on a basal lamina formed jointly by themselves and podocytes.
E: are in close proximity to the secondary processes of podocytes.

Learning Response A: Correct. The urinary space is that space between the visceral and parietal layers of Bowman's capsule. The visceral layer is composed of modified epithelial cells known as podocytes, and the parietal layer consists of simple squamous epithelium. One should remember that, unlike other fenestrated capillaries, those of the glomerulus have no diaphragms. Do not confuse this with the fact that filtration slits (formed by podocytes) do have diaphragms.

511. SUBJECT AREA: Urinary System

QUESTION: All of the following can help distinguish the thin segment of the loop of Henle from the vasa recta EXCEPT

A: the type of epithelial lining.
B: thickness of the wall.
C: the content of the lumen.
D: the appearance of the nuclei.
E: presence of fenestrae in the wall.

Learning Response A: Correct. Both structures are lined by simple squamous epithelium which adds to the difficulty in distinguishing between them in histological sections. Of all the choices listed above, the presence of erythrocytes in the lumen of the vasa recta would be the most useful clue in differentiating between these two components of the renal medulla.

512. SUBJECT AREA: Urinary System

QUESTION: In the figure below, the epithelium is best described as typical of

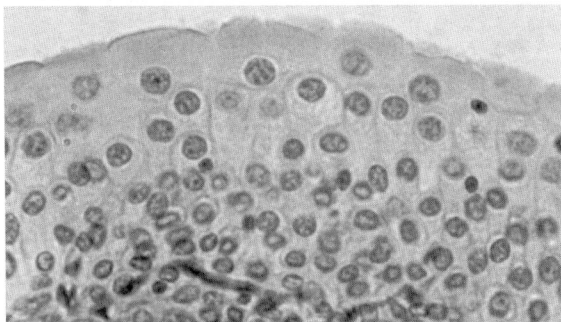

A: the urinary bladder.
B: the ureters.

C: the renal pelvis.

D: the minor calyces.

E: all the above structures.

Learning Response E: Correct. The epithelium shown is transitional epithelium which is found in all of the above structures.

513. SUBJECT AREA: Urinary System

QUESTION: The macula densa is characterized by all of the following EXCEPT

A: it, along with juxtaglomerular (JG) cells, forms the juxtaglomerular apparatus.

B: its cells are characterized as darkly staining, columnar cells with tightly packed nuclei.

C: it is found in close proximity to the urinary pole of the renal corpuscle.

D: it may send information on distal tubule fluid osmolality to the afferent arteriole.

E: it is a modified segment of cells in the wall of the distal tubule.

Learning Response C: Correct. The macula densa is a modified segment of the wall of the distal tubule. It is located at a point of close contact with the vascular pole of the renal corpuscle of its parent nephron. Although its function is not completely understood, the macula densa may play a role in transferring information on distal tubule fluid osmolality to the afferent arteriole. The macula densa and the JG cells form the juxtaglomerular apparatus.

514. SUBJECT AREA: Urinary System

QUESTION: After the renal artery divides in the hilum, blood circulating to the kidney flows through the

A: interlobar arteries, arcuate arteries, interlobular arteries, afferent arterioles.

B: interlobar arteries, interlobular arteries, arcuate arteries, afferent arterioles.

C: interlobular arteries, arcuate arteries, interlobar
arteries, afferent arterioles.

D: interlobular arteries, interlobar arteries, arcuate
arteries, afferent arterioles.

E: interlobar arteries, arcuate arteries, interlobular
arteries, efferent arterioles.

Learning Response A: Correct. The interlobar arteries are found between the renal pyramids and branch at the corticomedullary junction into the arcuate arteries. The arcuate arteries give rise to the interlobular arteries which flow through the cortex perpendicular to the renal capsule. The interlobular arteries give rise to the afferent arterioles which feed the glomerular capillary network. Blood then exits the glomerulus via the efferent arterioles which immediately branch to form a peritubular capillary network. Correspondingly, the vasa recta is a capillary network formed by branches of efferent arterioles associated with juxtamedullary nephrons. Blood returns via the venous system which is similarly labeled.

---

515. SUBJECT AREA: Urinary System

QUESTION: Which of the following associations is NOT correct?

A: loop of Henle—production of hypertonic urine

B: descending thick limb—similar in structure to the
proximal tubule

C: descending thin limb—freely permeable to water

D: ascending thin limb—freely permeable to water

E: ascending thick limb—active transport of chloride

Learning Response D: Correct. The loop of Henle is the structure which enables humans to produce a hypertonic urine. The descending thick limb, which is similar in structure to the proximal convoluted tubule, narrows to a width of 12 μm to become the thin descending limb which is composed of simple squamous epithelium and is freely permeable to water. Although both thin and thick ascending limbs are impermeable to water, the ascending thick limb is a site for active transport of chloride ions into the lumen; sodium ions follow passively. This active transport allows for the formation of a hypertonic medullary interstitium which is necessary for the ultimate formation of hypertonic urine.

516. SUBJECT AREA: Urinary System
QUESTION: A tumor originating in the epithelium of the bladder would most likely be a

A: squamous cell carcinoma.
B: tumor of skeletal muscle origin.
C: tumor of smooth muscle origin.
D: transitional cell carcinoma.
E: tumor of connective tissue origin.

Learning Response D: Correct. Ninety per cent of bladder tumors are derived from the epithelium. Transitional epithelium is also found in the calyces, pelvis and ureter.

517. SUBJECT AREA: Urinary System
QUESTION: The male urethra

A: is lined solely by transitional epithelium.
B: collects the secretions of the glands of Littré.
C: does not receive secretions from the prostate gland.
D: consists of bulbous and pendulous portions found within the prostate gland.
E: is characterized by all of the above responses.

Learning Response B: Correct. The male urethra is both a conduit for urine and semen. The prostatic portion is lined by transitional epithelium, while other portions may be lined with stratified squamous, stratified columnar, or pseudostratified columnar epithelium. The bulbous and pendulous portions of the urethra are found within the corpus spongiosum of the penis. Littré's glands are mucous glands found along the entire length of the urethra. The prostate is a glandular organ that produces a fluid that is secreted into the prostatic urethra during ejaculation and is a component of semen.

518. SUBJECT AREA: Urinary System
QUESTION: Renin

A: is released in response to a decrease in blood pressure.

B: is secreted by juxtaglomerular cells.

C: assists in the formation of an extremely potent vasoconstrictor.

D: release ultimately impacts on the absorption of sodium and chloride ions.

E: can be characterized by all of the above statements.

Learning Response E: Correct. Renin, secreted by JG cells, acts on a plasma protein, angiotensinogen, to produce angiotensin I, which is converted in the lung to angiontensin II, a potent vasoconstrictor which assists in the maintenance of blood pressure. In addition, angiotensin II also stimulates the release of aldosterone from the adrenal cortex. Aldosterone enhances the absorption of sodium and chloride ions from renal distal tubule cells.

519. SUBJECT AREA: Urinary System

QUESTION: Juxtamedullary nephrons are characterized by all of the following EXCEPT that they

A: play a key role in establishing the hypertonic gradient present in the medulla.

B: are fewer in number than cortical nephrons.

C: have very short Henle's loops.

D: are located near the corticomedullary junction.

E: participate in the processes of filtration, absorption and secretion.

Learning Response C: Correct. Juxtamedullary nephrons are found near the corticomedullary junction and have very long Henle's loops which penetrate deep into the renal medulla. This allows the thin limbs of these nephrons to play a major role in the formation of the gradient of hypertonicity in the medulla. Approximately one-seventh of all nephrons are of the juxtamedullary type; all nephrons participate in the processes of filtration, absorption and secretion.

520. SUBJECT AREA: Urinary System
      QUESTION: In the figure below, the cells

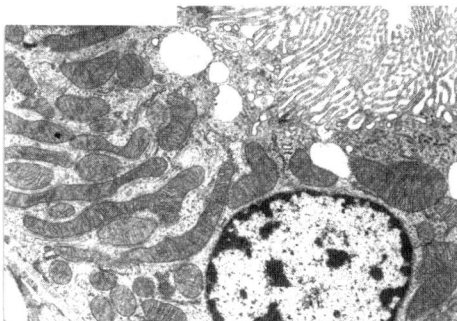

    A: form the parietal layer of Bowman's capsule.
    B: are cells of the proximal convoluted tubule.
    C: are mesangial cells.
    D: form the visceral layer of Bowman's capsule.
    E: are cells of the distal convoluted tubule.

Learning Response B: Correct. The cells are those of the proximal tubule, which are identified by the presence of microvilli at their apical surface organized into a brush border. None of the other choices has these structures arranged as a brush border.

521. SUBJECT AREA: Urinary System
      QUESTION: In regard to the formation of urine,

    A: the vasa recta further contribute to the osmotic gradient by active transport of sodium ions.
    B: the osmotic gradient is most pronounced in the kidney cortex.
    C: the osmotic gradient is formed solely by the vasa recta.
    D: the osmotic gradient ensures the formation of hypertonic urine.
    E: none of the above statements are correct.

Learning Response E: Correct. The loop of Henle forms an osmotic gradient in the medullary interstitium by the repetitive transport of sodium and chloride ions—the "countercurrent multiplier" system. The vasa recta, or straight vessels of the medullary region, do not contribute to the formation of the osmotic gradient. Although passive movement of sodium and water occurs in these vessels, no change in the interstitial osmolality is produced. This is the so-called "countercurrent exchange" system. Although the osmotic gradient is essential to the production of hypertonic urine, only hypotonic urine will be formed in the absence of antidiuretic hormone (vasopressin).

---

522. Subject Area: Urinary System
   Question: The glomerular basement membrane

   A: is a charge and size-selective barrier.
   B: secretes sodium into the glomerular filtrate.
   C: is unique in that it lacks proteoglycans.
   D: contains large amounts of type I collagen.
   E: is characterized by all of the above statements.

Learning Response A: Correct. The glomerular basement membrane consists of a central lamina densa bounded by a lighter lamina rara on either side. The membrane is both a mechanical and electrical barrier: type IV collagen in the lamina densa and negatively charged heparan sulfate in the lamina rara are important functional components.

---

523. Subject Area: Respiratory System
   Question: A function of the blood supply of the lamina propria of the conducting portion of the respiratory system is to

   A: warm the incoming air.
   B: supply the epithelium with eosinophils.
   C: carry away pathogens.
   D: attack viruses.
   E: detoxify the incoming air.

Learning Response A: Correct. A major function of the conducting portion of the respiratory system is to condition incoming air. The rich capillary network warms the air that enters the nasal and oral cavities.

524. SUBJECT AREA: Respiratory System

QUESTION: Alveoli are connected to one another by alveolar pores which are clinically relevant in that they allow

A: macrophages to attack bacteria.
B: for the spread of surfactant to all alveoli.
C: for the spread of infection to other alveoli.
D: eosinophils to migrate from one alveolus to another.
E: for the attachment of mast cells in allergic reactions.

Learning Response C: Correct. Bacteria can spread from one alveolus to another through the pores.

525. SUBJECT AREA: Respiratory System

QUESTION: Surfactant

A: is produced by type I pneumocytes.
B: decreases the surface tension at the epithelial-air interface.
C: is a component of the basement membrane of the alveolar epithelium.
D: is produced by alveolar macrophages.
E: coats the nasal epithelium.

Learning Response B: Correct. Surfactant secreted by type II alveolar cells onto alveolar surfaces is high in lipid content and functions to lower the surface tension along the alveoli.

526. SUBJECT AREA: Respiratory System

QUESTION: Bronchi

A: have plates of hyaline cartilage in their walls.
B: lack goblet cells.
C: lack cilia.
D: lack smooth muscle.

E: contain alveoli as part of their walls.

Learning Response A: Correct. The more proximal regions of the bronchi are similar in structure to the trachea. As the diameter of the bronchi decrease, the hyaline cartilage breaks up into plates of tissue.

527. SUBJECT AREA: Respiratory System
QUESTION: The primary function of the elastic fibers in the conducting and respiratory portions of the respiratory system is to

A: provide a scaffold for the organs.
B: provide flexibility and distensibilty of the organs.
C: prevent distension of the organ.
D: form a molecular sieve preventing the spread of pathogens.
E: support the lymphoid tissue found in many of the organs.

Learning Response B: Correct. Elastic fibers in the lamina propria of the conducting portion and in the interstitial tissue of the respiratory portion allow for distension and flexibility of the organs.

528. SUBJECT AREA: Respiratory System
QUESTION: What best describes the concentration of the elastic fibers in the conducting system?

A: Elastic fibers are randomly arranged and equally distributed throughout the system.
B: The nasal lamina propria contains the greatest amount of elastic fibers.
C: Because of the presence of cartilaginous rings, the trachea lacks elastic fibers.
D: The smaller the bronchiole, the greater the amount of elastic fibers.
E: Elastic fiber concentration is highest in the larynx.

Learning Response D: Correct. Elastic fiber concentrations are inversely proportional to the diameter of the conducting tube; the smallest bronchioles have the greatest concentration of elastic fibers.

---

529. SUBJECT AREA: Respiratory System

QUESTION: Hyaline cartilage provides structural support for all of the following components of the respiratory system EXCEPT the

A: larynx.
B: nasal region.
C: trachea.
D: bronchi.
E: bronchioles.

Learning Response E: Correct. As the diameter of the conducting tube decreases to form the bronchioles in the lung, hyaline cartilage in the walls of the tube is replaced by smooth muscle which provides support for those structures.

---

530. SUBJECT AREA: Respiratory System

QUESTION: In the figure below, identify the structure with the widest lumen.

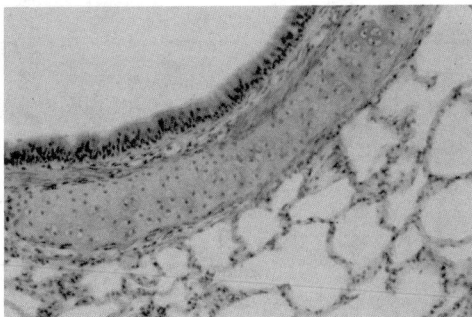

A: muscular bronchiole
B: alveolus
C: bronchus
D: respiratory bronchiole
E: trachea

Learning Response C: Correct. The presence of alveoli at the lower right of the image confirms that this is a section through the lung, effectively eliminating the trachea from consideration. Bronchi are lined with pseudostratified epithelium and have plates of hyaline cartilage in their outer walls. None of the other structures in the lung has these tissues.

---

531. SUBJECT AREA: Respiratory System

QUESTION: What is the main significance of the absence of mucus secreting cells and the presence of ciliated cells in the bronchioles?

A: Particulate matter in the bronchioles can be swept toward the more distally located mucus.

B: Mucus is prevented from accumulating in more distal areas of the system.

C: The more distal regions no longer require a surface tension-reducing layer of mucus.

D: Cilia assist in the movement of surfactant material through the bronchioles and alveoli.

E: Cilia are necessary to aid in the migration of macrophages from the bronchioles to the alveoli.

Learning Response B: Correct. Mucus would accumulate in the alveoli if the cells of the terminal and respiratory bronchioles lacked cilia.

---

532. SUBJECT AREA: Respiratory System

QUESTION: Nonciliated Clara cells are located in the _____ and function

A: alveoli / in surface tension reduction by surfactant secretion.

B: trachea / in glycogen secretion.

C: bronchioles / to protect the lining by secretion of glycosaminoglycans.

D: bronchi / as a stem cell population.

E: nasal mucosa / by secreting enzymes which degrade odoriferous chemicals.

Learning Response C: Correct. Noncilated cells which form part of the epithelium in the terminal bronchioles contain secretory granules and secrete glycosaminoglycans which may protect the lining of the tube. There is also evidence that Clara cells produce a lipid material which can reduce surface tension in the bronchioles. This substance is different from surfactant secreted by type II alveolar cells.

---

533. SUBJECT AREA: Respiratory System

QUESTION: All of the following types of cells are found in the epithelial lining of the respiratory system EXCEPT

A: brush cells.
B: small granule neuroendocrine cells.
C: stem cells in the basal layers.
D: surfactant secreting cells.
E: steroid hormone secreting cells.

Learning Response E: Correct. Steroid-secreting cells are absent from the respiratory system. Small granule cells secrete a neuroendocrine substance which may integrate the mucous and serous secretory functions of the epithelial cells. Brush cells have numerous apically located microvilli and nerve fiber terminations at their basal surface. Type II pneumocytes secrete surfactant.

---

534. SUBJECT AREA: Respiratory System

QUESTION: The major types of cells located in the alveoli include

A: type I and II alveolar cells, endothelial cells, macrophages and interstitial cells.
B: brush cells and nonciliated Clara cells.
C: basal cells, endothelial cells, type I alveolar cells, macrophages.
D: mucus-secreting cells, type II alveolar cells, endothelial cells and macrophages.
E: endothelial cells, type I alveolar cells and macrophages.

Learning Response A: Correct. Type I and type II alveolar cells (also known as type I and type II pneumocytes) constitute the lining cells of the alveoli. Macrophages are located in the interstitial tissue along with fibroblasts and leukocytes. Macrophages can also move along the epithelial lining.

535. SUBJECT AREA: Respiratory System
QUESTION: Which of the following best describes the blood-air barrier?

A: The presence of a thick basement membrane in the alveoli.
B: The presence of a fused basal lamina between two populations of epithelial cells.
C: A layer of surfactant-coated type I and type II alveolar cells.
D: The population of macrophages in the interstitial tissue.
E: A thick layer of mucus along the surface of the alveoli.

Learning Response B: Correct. The basal laminae of the endothelial cells and the type I alveolar cells fuse to form a thin band of tissue between the two types of epithelial cells.

536. SUBJECT AREA: Respiratory System
QUESTION: The trachea

A: is lined by pseudostratified ciliated epithelium containing goblet cells.
B: contains C-shaped rings of hyaline cartilage to prevent its lumen from collapsing.
C: has a bundle of smooth muscle and fibroelastic tissue in its posterior wall.
D: has glands in the lamina propria.
E: exhibits all of the above features.

Learning Response E: Correct. The trachea extends from the base of the larynx to the primary bronchi and possesses all of the histological characteristics presented in the question.

537. SUBJECT AREA: Respiratory System
    QUESTION: In the larynx,

> A: the epithelium changes to the stratified squamous
>   type along the true vocal cords.
> B: the vocalis muscle is involuntary smooth muscle.
> C: mucous and serous glands are absent.
> D: the more caudal false vocal cords are covered by
>   respiratory epithelium.
> E: the epiglottis is located just below the true vocal
>   cords.

Learning Response A: Correct. The true vocal cords are covered by stratified squamous epithelium under which is the vocalis muscle which is striated skeletal or voluntary muscle.

538. SUBJECT AREA: Respiratory System
    QUESTION: The large venous plexuses (swell bodies) in the lamina
    propria of the nasal conchae

> A: can become engorged with blood which decreases
>   the flow of air.
> B: can alternate the flow of air from one nasal fossa to
>   the other.
> C: assist in the recovery of the respiratory epithelium
>   from desiccation.
> D: have features listed by choices A, B and C above.
> E: exhibit features given in A and B above.

Learning Response D: Correct. The alternate swelling and receding of the venous plexuses allow air to cycle from one side of the nasal cavity to the other. These periodic occlusions of air flow are important to prevent drying of the nasal epithelium.

539. SUBJECT AREA: Respiratory System
    QUESTION: Defects in the gene encoding the protein dynein

A: would result in the immotile cilia syndrome (Kartagener's syndrome).
B: would result in the accumulation of mucus in the alveoli.
C: would produce an accumulation of mucus in the nasal passages.
D: probably would result in all of the above examples.
E: probably would result in only two of the above examples.

Learning Response D: Correct. Dynein is the protein responsible for the movement of cilia and a defect or deficiency in this protein would allow mucus to accumulate in several areas of the respiratory tract.

---

540. SUBJECT AREA: Respiratory System
QUESTION: All of the following are functions of pulmonary macrophages EXCEPT

A: phagocytosis of bacteria.
B: secretion of enzymes, especially collagenase and lysozyme.
C: ingestion of carbon and other particulate material.
D: functioning as antigen presenting cells as part of pulmonary immune responses.
E: liberation of carbon dioxide by the action of the enzyme carbonic anhydrase.

Learning Response E: Correct. Pulmonary macrophages have several important functions. However, the liberation of carbon dioxide is a function of the red blood cells in the alveolar capillaries.

---

541. SUBJECT AREA: Respiratory System
QUESTION: The tissue associated with the exchange of oxygen and carbon dioxide is

A: respiratory epithelium.
B: transitional epithelium.

> *C:* pseudostratified epithelium with cilia and goblet cells.
> *D:* simple squamous epithelium.
> *E:* stratified squamous epithelium.

Learning Response D: Correct. Type I alveolar cells line the alveoli and as a tissue they constitute simple squamous epithelium through which gases are exchanged.

---

542. SUBJECT AREA: Respiratory System
QUESTION: Type II alveolar cells (great alveolar cells)

> *A:* are also called dust cells.
> *B:* secrete material which decreases the surface tension of the alveolar wall.
> *C:* are derived from monocytes.
> *D:* are the most common cell type lining the bronchioles.
> *E:* are involved in the exchange of gases.

Learning Response B: Correct. Type II alveolar cells (type II pneumocytes) secrete pulmonary surfactant which lowers surface tension so that the walls of the alveoli do not adhere upon exhalation. Type II alveolar cells arise from the same stem cells as type I alveolar cells and cover only 3% of the alveolar surface, but play no role in gas exchange. Alveolar macrophages, also known as dust cells, are derived from monocytes.

---

543. SUBJECT AREA: Respiratory System
QUESTION: The conducting portion of the respiratory system consists of all of the following EXCEPT

> *A:* alveolar duct.
> *B:* trachea.
> *C:* bronchi.
> *D:* larynx.
> *E:* nares.

Learning Response A: Correct. Distal to the respiratory bronchioles are the alveolar ducts which are considered to be part of the respiratory portion of the system since gas exchange can occur there.

---

544. SUBJECT AREA: Respiratory System
       QUESTION: A terminal bronchiole

         A: contains plates of hyaline cartilage in its wall.
         B: lacks goblet cells.
         C: is lined with pseudostratified epithelium.
         D: lacks smooth muscle.
         E: contains alveoli.

Learning Response B: Correct. Mucus secreting goblet cells are absent from the terminal bronchioles while ciliated cells remain a part of the epithelial lining.

---

545. SUBJECT AREA: Respiratory System
       QUESTION: Which of the following statements about the
                 respiratory system is NOT correct?

         A: Bronchi can be distinguished from bronchioles by
            the presence of cartilaginous plates in the bronchi.
         B: Alveolar outpouches are characteristic of
            respiratory bronchioles.
         C: The epiglottis is completely covered by stratified
            squamous epithelium on both surfaces.
         D: Lymphoid nodules can be present in the wall of the
            bronchi.
         E: Lamellar bodies can be found in the cytoplasm of
            type II alveolar cells.

Learning Response C: Correct. The epiglottis has stratified squamous epithelium on its lingual surface which is replaced by ciliated pseudostratified columnar epithelium on its laryngeal surface.

---

546. SUBJECT AREA: Respiratory System

QUESTION: The conducting part of the respiratory system contains all of the following EXCEPT

A: neuroendocrine cells.
B: plasma cells.
C: bone.
D: skeletal muscle.
E: heart failure cells.

Learning Response E: Correct. In congestive heart failure, erythrocytes pass into the alveoli where they are ingested by alveolar macrophages. Hemoglobin is metabolized within the macrophages to hemosiderin which gives these "heart failure cells" a brownish color when they are stained for iron pigment.

547. SUBJECT AREA: Respiratory System
QUESTION: One of the effects of an asthmatic attack is

A: the contraction of bronchiolar smooth muscle causing difficulty breathing.
B: an increase in the production of collagen by fibroblasts.
C: a decrease in the concentration of surfactant along the alveoli.
D: an increase in the numbers of lymphoid nodules.
E: a decrease in the numbers of alveolar macrophages.

Learning Response A: Correct. The smooth muscle layer of the bronchioles is better developed than that of the bronchi. Increased airway resistance in asthma is believed to be the result of the contraction of bronchiolar smooth muscle.

548. SUBJECT AREA: Respiratory System
QUESTION: Antibodies to which of the following intermediate filament proteins would be useful in differentiating squamous cell carcinoma of the lung?

A: desmin
B: vimentin
C: lamin

D: cytokeratin

E: glial fibrillary acidic protein (GFAP)

Learning Response D: Correct. Squamous epithelial cells have cytokeratin as their type of cytoplasmic intermediate filament protein. Reaction of pathological tissue with antibodies against this protein is helpful in diagnosis of epithelial derived carcinomas. Vimentin can be found in mesenchymal cells; desmin in muscle cells; GFAP in glial cells such as astrocytes; lamin in the fibrous lamina of the nucleus.

---

549. SUBJECT AREA: Respiratory System

QUESTION: The lungs of individuals afflicted with emphysema are greatly dilated and exhibit an inability to expel air. This condition is most likely the result of

A: a breakdown of the elastic fibers in the lungs.

B: an increase in collagen content in the lungs.

C: a depletion of the fibroblasts in the pulmonary interstitium.

D: increased phagocytic activity of fibroblasts.

E: enhanced immune reactions in the lungs.

Learning Response A: Correct. During inhalation, the elastic fibers are stretched by expansion. The retraction of the lungs in exhalation is the result of the reduction in the tension on the elastic fibers. Increased elastase activity in the lungs of emphysematmous patients causes the destruction of elastin and results in a loss in the ability of the lungs to reduce their size on exhalation. It has been suggested that cigarette smoke contributes to the pathogenesis of emphysema by increased elastase activity as well as decreased activity of protective proteases (such as antitrypsin).

---

550. SUBJECT AREA: Respiratory System

QUESTION: The respiratory bronchiole is so named because it

A: contains numerous alveolar macrophages.

B: contains sites for the exchange of gases.

C: is lined with respiratory epithelium.

D: is lined with ciliated cells.

> *E:* is associated with the secretion of surfactant.

Learning Response B: Correct. Gas exchange can occur at sites along the wall of the respiratory bronchiole, and this function gives rise to the name. The structure is lined with ciliated simple cuboidal epithelium.

---

551. SUBJECT AREA: Respiratory System

QUESTION: Type I alveolar cells have all of the following features EXCEPT that they

A: constitute less than 25% of the alveolar surface.

B: can exhibit pinocytotic vesicles which may function in surfactant turnover.

C: are so attenuated that they are best seen by electron microscopy.

D: have occluding junctions between adjacent cells to prevent leakage of tissue fluid into the alveoli.

E: have their major organelles clustered near the nucleus in order to reduce the thickness of the blood-air barrier.

Learning Response A: Correct. The type I cells make up approximately 97% of the alveolar surface while type II cells constitute the remaining 3%.

---

552. SUBJECT AREA: Respiratory System

QUESTION: The type of pulmonary blood vessel which would be found in the adventitia of the bronchioles is the

A: capillary.

B: pulmonary metarteriole.

C: pulmonary artery.

D: pulmonary vein.

E: pulmonary venules.

Learning Response C: Correct. Pulmonary arteries accompany the bronchial tree and are located within the adventitia of the bronchi and bronchioles.

553. SUBJECT AREA: Organs of Special Sense

QUESTION: The crista ampullaris sends information to the central nervous system on

A: angular acceleration.
B: linear acceleration.
C: tilt of the head.
D: pitch of sound.
E: amplitude of sound waves.

Learning Response A: Correct. Endolymphatic fluid in the semicircular canals stimulates the hair cells of the cristae in response to rotational movements of the head or angular acceleration. Linear acceleration and the position of the head in space are sensed by the macula in the inner ear, and sound is detected by cells in the organ of Corti in the cochlea.

554. SUBJECT AREA: Organs of Special Sense

QUESTION: The major cytoplasmic component of the pillar cells in the organ of Corti is

A: mitochondria.
B: microfilaments.
C: rough endoplasmic reticulum.
D: intermediate filaments.
E: microtubules.

Learning Response E: Correct. The pillar cells support the hair cells of the organ of Corti, and the large number of microtubules, which are aggregated into bundles, impart a stiffness to these cells.

555. SUBJECT AREA: Organs of Special Sense

QUESTION: The optic nerve is composed of axons from which of the following cell types?

A: bipolar cells
B: rod cells
C: cone cells

D: amacrine cells

E: ganglion cells

Learning Response E: Correct. The ganglion cells are located in one of the innermost retinal layers and send their axons to the optic nerve. The rods and cones are the receptor cells, and the bipolar cells and amacrine cells are neurons with cell bodies located in the inner nuclear layer.

---

556. SUBJECT AREA: Organs of Special Sense

QUESTION: Which of the layers of the cornea is responsible for maintaining its transparency?

A: endothelium

B: stroma

C: Descemet's membrane

D: Bowman's membrane

E: All the layers of the cornea function to keep it transparent.

Learning Response A: Correct. The endothelium and the outer epithelium function in keeping the cornea transparent. Both layers are capable of transporting ions and water to maintain the stroma in a relatively dry state.

---

557. SUBJECT AREA: Organs of Special Sense

QUESTION: Cells which rest on the basilar membrane of the organ of Corti include

A: inner phalangeal cells.

B: inner pillar cells.

C: outer pillar cells.

D: inner hair cells.

E: choices A, B and C above.

Learning Response E: Correct. Neither the inner hair cells nor the outer hair cells rest on the basilar membrane but are cradled by the phalangeal cells. Pillar cells line the triangular space (the inner tunnel) between the inner and outer hair cells.

558. SUBJECT AREA: Organs of Special Sense

QUESTION: Damage to the blood vessels that form the choriocapillary layer would most likely result in

A: degeneration of the optic nerve.
B: degeneration of the receptor cells.
C: chromatolysis in the bipolar neurons.
D: depletion of ganglion cells.
E: disruption of the inner limiting membrane.

Learning Response B: Correct. The choriocapillary vessels provide metabolites to the outermost layers of the retina, those which include the rods and cones. Any interruption in the blood supply would have damaging effects on the receptor cells. The inner layers of the retina are supplied by the central artery which enters the retina from the optic disc, a structure which carries optic nerve fibers.

559. SUBJECT AREA: Organs of Special Sense

QUESTION: The histological features of the lacrimal gland closely resemble those of the

A: sebaceous gland.
B: sublingual gland.
C: endocrine pancreas.
D: parotid gland.
E: eyelid glands of Zeis.

Learning Response D: Correct. The acini of the lacrimal gland are of the serous type and resemble those of the parotid gland. The glands of Zeis in the eyelid are modified sebaceous glands which empty into the follicles of the eyelashes and as such resemble the more common type of sebaceous glands found in the skin. A system of ducts drains the lacrimal gland and, therefore, it has no similarity to the ductless endocrine glands.

560. SUBJECT AREA: Organs of Special Sense

QUESTION: All of the following are features of the olfactory epithelium EXCEPT

A: the receptor cells have cilia that are parallel to the surface.

B: junctional complexes attach the supporting cells to the receptor cells.

C: basal cell nuclei are located near the basement membrane.

D: odors have to be dissolved in mucus for sensation to occur.

E: the olfactory cells can be classified as multipolar neurons.

Learning Response E: Correct. The olfactory receptor cells are bipolar neurons, the axons of which are directed toward the central nervous system.

561. SUBJECT AREA: Organs of Special Sense

QUESTION: The epithelium of the lens is unique in that

A: its basement membrane, the lens capsule, is located at the surface of the structure.

B: capillaries can be found between the cuboidal epithelial cells.

C: the epithelial cells lack cell to cell junctions.

D: it contains an abundance of free nerve endings.

E: it lacks a basement membrane.

Learning Response A: Correct. The lens capsule coats the outer surface of the epithelial cells and consists mainly of type IV collagen and glycoprotein. As such, it has a number of features in common with basement membrane associated with other types of epithelial cells. Capillaries are usually not located within an epithelium such as that found in the lens. An exception to this is the stria vascularis of the cochlea which does contain blood vessels. The lens epithelial cells have communicating or gap junctions.

562. SUBJECT AREA: Organs of Special Sense

QUESTION: A blockage in the canal of Schlemm would most likely result in

A: an increase in intraocular pressure.

> *B:* increased amounts of aqueous humor in the anterior chamber.
> *C:* a clinical condition known as glaucoma.
> *D:* eventual blindness if allowed to remain uncorrected.
> *E:* all of the above possibilities.

Learning Response E: Correct. Any interruption in the drainage of aqueous humor by the canal of Schlemm and the scleral venous system can have severe detrimental effects for the individual if left untreated.

563. SUBJECT AREA: Organs of Special Sense
   QUESTION: Contraction of the ciliary muscles results in

> *A:* an enlarged pupillary opening.
> *B:* a smaller pupillary opening.
> *C:* a relaxation in the zonule and a thicker lens.
> *D:* tension of the zonule causing the lens to thicken.
> *E:* a condition called a cataract leading to an increase in lens opacity.

Learning Response C: Correct. Contraction of the ciliary muscles displaces the choroid and ciliary bodies forward which relieves the tension on the zonule fibers and results in a thickening of the lens as part of a process known as accommodation. Cataracts are the result of an accumulation of pigment in the lens fibers, and this renders the fibers less transparent.

564. SUBJECT AREA: Organs of Special Sense
   QUESTION: Infections in the upper respiratory tract often lead to middle ear infections resulting from passage of bacteria through the

> *A:* tympanic membrane.
> *B:* auditory (Eustachian) tube.
> *C:* oval window.
> *D:* round window.
> *E:* cochlear duct.

Learning Response B: Correct. The middle ear cavity communicates with the pharynx by means of the auditory tube which can serve as a passageway for infections. The oval and round windows and cochlear duct are located in the inner ear.

---

565. SUBJECT AREA: Organs of Special Sense
QUESTION: The histological features of the cristae ampullares and the maculae of the saccule and utricle are similar EXCEPT

A: for the presence of a gelatinous glycoprotein membrane associated with the cristae.
B: for the type of receptor cells.
C: that the cristae are bathed by perilymph while the maculae are nourished by endolymph.
D: for the presence of calcium carbonate crystals associated with the maculae.
E: that the receptor cells of the maculae lack stereocilia.

Learning Response D: Correct. The receptor cells or hair cells of both structures have stereocilia which are embedded in a gelatinous membrane of glycoprotein. Associated with this membrane in the maculae are crystals of calcium carbonate called otoliths or otoconia which can help distinguish between the maculae and the cristae. Both cristae and maculae are bathed by endolymph, and the hair cells, which are similar in both areas, have stereocilia at their surface.

---

566. SUBJECT AREA: Organs of Special Sense
QUESTION: The bony labyrinth consists of

A: the vestibule, cochlea and semicircular canals.
B: the malleus, incus and stapes.
C: the utricle and saccule.
D: connective tissue bathed by endolymph.
E: the endolymphatic duct and sac.

Learning Response A: Correct. The three semicircular canals, the bony cochlea and the vestibule are all components of the bony labyrinth within which is housed the membranous labyrinth consisting of the saccule, utricle, endolymphatic duct and sac, ducts within the semicircular canals and scala media or cochlear duct.

---

567. SUBJECT AREA: Organs of Special Sense
QUESTION: Of importance to the sensation of hearing is that

    A: the hair cells rest directly on the basilar membrane.
    B: fluid within the scalae remains static.
    C: the stereocilia of the outer hair cells are embedded in the tectorial membrane.
    D: the scala vestibuli and scala tympani are not connected to each other.
    E: the hair cells possess a single, non-motile cilium.

Learning Response C: Correct. Shearing forces against the stereocilia of the outer hair cells in the tectorial membrane cause displacement of the stereocilia and open gated calcium channels in the receptor cells initiating the process of signal transduction leading to the generation of action potentials in the auditory nerve fibers. Fluid in the scalae is set in motion by the movements of sound waves transmitted from the footplate of the stapes to the oval window. The scala vestibuli and scala tympani are connected to each other at the apex of the cochlea, the helicotrema.

---

568. SUBJECT AREA: Organs of Special Sense
QUESTION: All of the following receptors detect pressure, vibration and touch EXCEPT

    A: Meissner's corpuscles.
    B: Pacinian corpuscles.
    C: Ruffini's endings.
    D: Golgi tendon organs.
    E: Merkel's discs.

Learning Response D: Correct. Golgi tendon organs are encapsulated proprioceptors associated with collagen fibers in myotendinous junctions.

569. SUBJECT AREA: Organs of Special Sense
QUESTION: All of the following are enclosed within the connective tissue capsules of muscle spindles EXCEPT

A: intrafusal muscle fibers.
B: sensory nerve fibers.
C: nuclear chain fibers.
D: extrafusal muscle fibers.
E: nuclear bag fibers.

Learning Response D: Correct. The large muscle fibers outside of the encapsulated muscle spindles are called extrafusal fibers. There are two types of intrafusal fibers, those within the connective tissue capsule: nuclear chain fibers and nuclear bag fibers named for their arrangements of myonuclei. The nuclear bag fibers have centrally located clusters of nuclei, and the nuclear chain fibers have linearly dispersed nuclei. Each of these two types of intrafusal fibers have different morphologies of their afferent terminations.

570. SUBJECT AREA: Organs of Special Sense
QUESTION: In regard to the sensation of taste,

A: taste buds are restricted to the surface of the tongue.
B: the major receptor cell is the type III cell which contains numerous vesicles.
C: taste buds are located in the connective tissue of the lingual papillae.
D: receptor cells in taste buds are one of two general cell types in that structure.
E: chemicals at the surface of the tongue must diffuse through the epithelial cells into the connective tissue in order to be detected.

Learning Response B: Correct. The vesicles within type III cells are thought to be synaptic vesicles. The proximity of dendritic neuronal processes to the accumulation of vesicles provides circumstantial evidence that type II cells are receptor cells. Taste buds are not confined to the tongue, but are also found in the soft palate and epiglottis and are located within the epithelium of the lingual surface. Four different types of cells have been identified in taste buds: two types of support cells, receptor cells and relatively undifferentiated basal cells. Chemicals enter the taste pore, an opening in the taste bud, and are in direct contact with the receptor cells.

571. SUBJECT AREA: Organs of Special Sense
QUESTION: In reference to the iris,

> A: the sphincter muscle is arranged in a circular pattern at the iridial margin.
> B: pigmented epithelium covers the anterior surface.
> C: the dilator muscle consists of a mixture of smooth and skeletal fibers.
> D: melanocytes in the stroma account for its coloration.
> E: choices A and D only are correct.

Learning Response E: Correct. As a result of its circular arrangement, the sphincter muscle closes the pupillary opening. The presence of melanocytes in the iridial stroma imparts color to the structure, the more cells the darker the color. The pigmented epithelium is located on the posterior aspect of the iris, and the dilator, like the sphincter muscle, consists only of smooth muscle fibers.

572. SUBJECT AREA: Organs of Special Sense
QUESTION: The major support cells of the retina are

> A: Müller cells.
> B: amacrine cells.
> C: horizontal cells.
> D: ganglion cells.
> E: bipolar cells.

Learning Response A: Correct. Müller cells extend from the inner to the outer limiting membrane and are the principal supporting cells of the retina. The other cells in the list are neuronal cells.

573. SUBJECT AREA: Organs of Special Sense
QUESTION: All of the following are true about the fovea EXCEPT

> *A:* the bipolar and ganglion cells are displaced toward the periphery of the area.
> *B:* that it consists of loosely packed receptor cells.
> *C:* the cone cells are elongated, and light falls directly on the receptor cells.
> *D:* vision is much sharper in the fovea than in other areas of the retina.
> *E:* in the center of the fovea the retina is thin.

Learning Response B: Correct. Cone cells in the fovea of the retina are closely packed together as a result of their elongated shape contributing to the increase in visual acuity of the area.

574. SUBJECT AREA: Organs of Special Sense
QUESTION: A diet deficient in vitamin A most likely

> *A:* results in seriously impaired color vision.
> *B:* increases difficulties in older individuals in driving at night.
> *C:* results in opacity of the cornea.
> *D:* increases membrane disk calcium ion concentration when the receptor cells are exposed to light.
> *E:* would have all of the above effects.

Learning Response B: Correct. Rhodopsin, the visual pigment of rods, consists of an aldehyde of vitamin A bound to protein. Rods are sensitive to low levels of illumination, and any deficit in vitamin A would impair the ability of individuals to drive at night. Bleaching of the visual pigment upon exposure to light increases the calcium ion concentration in the membrane disks under optimum levels of vitamin A.

575. SUBJECT AREA: Organs of Special Sense
QUESTION: In the discrimination of the frequency of sound waves,

A: the basilar membrane is maximally displaced at different positions along its length.

B: low frequency sound waves are detected near the apex of the cochlea.

C: high frequency sound waves are detected near the oval window.

D: the width of the basilar membrane is important for this function.

E: all of the above choices are correct.

Learning Response E: Correct. The stiffness of the basilar membrane is important in frequency discrimination. The stiff, narrow basilar membrane is maximally displaced near the oval window by high frequency waves and farther along its length by lower frequencies. The basilar membrane is most flexible at the helicotrema.

576. SUBJECT AREA: Organs of Special Sense
    QUESTION: The stria vascularis has all of the following features EXCEPT

A: that it contributes to the ionic composition of perilymph.

B: that it is located at the outer margin of the scala media (cochlear duct).

C: that it is a vascularized epithelium.

D: that its marginal cells have infoldings of their basal plasmalemma.

E: marginal cells have numerous basally located mitochondria.

Learning Response A: Correct. The marginal cells of the stria vascularis, which have all of the features of ion transporting cells, contribute to the ionic composition of endolymph which flows within the scala media.

577. SUBJECT AREA: Organs of Special Sense

QUESTION: Identify the structure shown in the figure below.

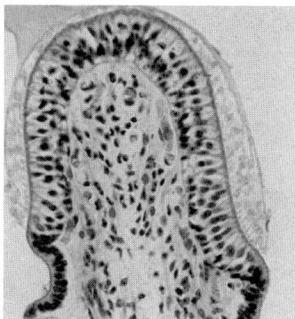

A: crista ampullaris
B: stria vascularis
C: organ of Corti
D: macula utriculi
D: spiral ganglion

Learning Response A: Correct. The ridges of neurosensory epithelium in the ampullae of the semicircular canals function in sensing movements caused by angular acceleration. The ridges or cristae contain two types of sensory cells along with support cells. Choices B, C and E are located in the cochlea. The maculae of the vestibule contain otoliths which are in contact with the stereocilia of the receptor cells. The otoliths are darkly stained by routine histological methods. The cristae lack otoliths.

Index

Numbers after index entries represent
question numbers.

A band, 210, 213
Accommodation, 563
Acetylcholine receptors, 189, 202
Acidophilia, 5
Acid phosphatase, 15, 125
Acinar cells, 423, 425, 428, 431
Acromegaly, 342
Acrosomal lysosomal enzymes, 454
ACTH, 84, 364, 366, 378
Actin
    amino acid sequence, 199
    binding, 202
    cytokinesis and, 17
    localization, 37
    microfilaments, 22, 29, 46, 56, 63,
        213, 413
    in skeletal muscle cells, 199
    synthesis, 27
Addison's disease, 370, 380
Adenohypophysis, 345, 358
Adenoma, benign somatotrophic, 342
ADH. See Antidiuretic hormone (ADH)
Adipocytes, 104, 107
Adipose tissue
    characteristics, 111
    functions, 109
    multilocular, 106, 113
Adrenal gland
    ACTH effects on, 364
    cortex
        cells, 362, 367
        fetal, 368
        insufficiency, 380
        stimulation, 378
        zona fasciculata, 386
    hyperfunction, 371
    insufficiency, 370
    medulla
        cells, 75, 364

chromaffin cells, 369, 372
    tumors of, 380
    zona fasciculata, 360, 364, 387
    zona glomerulosa, 387
    zona reticularis, 364, 387
Aging, morphological changes, 384
Albinism, 333
Aldosterone, 365, 383, 518
Allergic reactions, 95, 307
Alveolar cells, 540, 541, 551
Alveolar duct, 543
Alveoli, 524, 534, 539, 545
Amacrine cells, 555
Ameloblasts, 402
Amino acids, 82, 87
Ammonium sulfide, 15
Amylase, 421
Anchoring fibrils, 83
Androgen-binding protein, 445
Androgens, ovarian, 466
Aneurysm, 279
Angiosarcoma, 267
Angiotensin II, 508, 518
Angstrom, 4
Antibody/antibodies
    binding to myosin, 190
    to intermediate filament proteins,
        548
    secondary labeled, 9
Antidiuretic hormone (ADH; vaso-
        pressin)
    functions, 347, 354
    hypothalamo-hypophyseal neuronal
        tract and, 357
    papillary ducts and, 504
    secretion, 349
Antigen presenting cells (APCs), 300,
        336, 396
Antigens, 8
Antitrypsin, 549
Antrum, 464, 497
Aorta, 289